G000056947

A Special Issue of
Aphasiology

Computers and aphasia: Their role in the treatment of aphasia and the lives of people with aphasia

Edited by

Brian Petheram
Frenchay Hospital, Bristol, UK

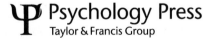 Psychology Press
Taylor & Francis Group

Published in 2004 by Psychology Press Ltd
27 Church Road, Hove, East Sussex, BN3 2FA
www.psypress.co.uk

Simultaneously published in the USA and Canada
by Taylor & Francis Inc.
29 West 35th Street, New York, NY 10001, USA

Psychology Press is part of the Taylor & Francis Group
© 2004 by Psychology Press Ltd

British Library Cataloguing in Publication Data
A catalogue record for this book is available from the British Library

ISBN 1-84169-977-2 (hbk)
ISSN 0268-7038

This book is also a special issue of the journal *Aphasiology* and forms issue 3 of
Volume 18 (2004).

Cover design by Leigh Hurlock
Typeset in the UK by DP Photosetting, Aylesbury, Bucks
Printed in the UK by Hobbs the Printer, Totton, Hants.

APHASIOLOGY

Volume 18   Number 3   March 2004

CONTENTS

APHASIOLOGY, 2004, *18* (3), 187–191

Editorial

Computers and aphasia:
A means of delivery and a delivery of means

Brian Petheram

University of the West of England and Frenchay Hospital, Bristol, UK

The idea of a special issue of *Aphasiology* devoted to the role of computers set off several trains of thought. It is some years since the last special issue on this topic and much has changed in the field since then. However it could be argued that computers as such are merely delivery mechanisms for therapy, and that their use is so commonplace that it is no longer a defining factor in a study. Certainly the use of computers in this field now has a long history; from early experiments with programmed instruction machines borrowed from language laboratories (Costello, 1977), through the series of studies by Katz, Nagy, and Tong beginning in 1982 that many would recognise as being the birth of the modern era of computer use in aphasia therapy. From the late 1980s through the 1990s many aphasia conferences would have a session devoted to papers on the use of computers. More recently it has been the case that many studies reported both in this journal and at conferences only mention in passing that computers were used, and focus on other aspects of the work.

However the role of information technology in the lives of individuals, organisations, and societies has been transformed over the last few years and the ways in which computers are used in aphasia therapy are beginning to reflect this. Rather than being deployed simply as a more efficient delivery mechanism, which essentially automates what had been done by human agents, computers are now also being used in ways that support activities which would not have been feasible without them. The papers in this special issue report on the use of computers from a range of perspectives: innovative ways of using computers for treatment; critical appraisals of their role and efficacy in aphasia rehabilitation; and ways in which computers can be used to enhance the daily lives of people with aphasia.

COMPUTERS AND TREATMENT

The two papers in this special issue on this topic, Mortley et al. and Doesborgh et al., exemplify the ways in which the use of computers can help to implement theories about good practice in aphasia therapy. Multicue, reported in Doesborgh et al., is interesting in that it engages the person with aphasia as a partner in treatment. It does this by allowing the user to experience the effect of several cueing strategies for naming, and by supporting the user in evaluating which strategy or strategies are most useful to him or her. Thus the

Address correspondence to: Brian Petheram, Speech & Language Therapy Research Unit, Frenchay Hospital, Bristol, UK. Email: brian@speech-therapy.org.uk

© 2004 Psychology Press Ltd

http://www.tandf.co.uk/journals/pp/02687038.html   DOI: 10.1080/02687030444000020

outcome of the treatment and the impact on the impairment are effected by a combination of the aphasiologist's knowledge of cueing theories and the client's own knowledge, preferences, strengths, and weaknesses. The computer is used to present the materials and, after an initial period with the therapist, the client uses the system more independently.

Mortley et al. report on a study that combines a leading edge use of technology with an implementation of theories about the necessity of tailoring therapy to the needs of the individual. No face-to-face treatment took place in this study. The computer was installed in the client's home and then all subsequent delivery and modification of the materials was implemented via the Internet, the client undertaking the exercises independently. This mode of delivery has huge potential for facilitating service delivery, particularly to clients in remote areas. However this study also addresses the issue of the quality of therapy delivered. Many earlier computer-based therapy systems relied on pre-defined exercises and some were relatively inflexible. The system developed by Mortley et al. can be tailored to the needs of individual clients by the therapist, without any need for either a visit to the client's home or any assistance from a computer specialist.

Both these studies show how computers can be used to deliver high-quality theory-based treatments in a way that engages the client and is cost effective in terms of service delivery. They are examples of how the use of computers can add value to treatment programmes.

DOES IT WORK?

If there ever was such a thing as a "honeymoon period" for the use of computers in this field, it is now long past and rightly so. There is a growing body of work that seeks to look behind the superficial glamour of the technology and ask hard questions about whether it works; for whom might it work; and what, if any is its role.

Wallesch and Johannsen-Horbach have reviewed a selection of studies, and conclude that while computer-based therapy may have some advantages, there may be some drawbacks in relation to potential "strain and burden" on the relationship between patient and partner in home-based situations. They call for a randomised controlled trial to evaluate the effectiveness of the computer component in treatment and its effect size.

Wertz and Katz focus on treatment outcomes and use a five phase model to classify and evaluate studies in computer-provided treatment of aphasia. Most of the studies Wertz and Katz found are in the very early phases, and they conclude that most studies have focused on efficacy and that different types of study in the phase 4 or 5 mode are needed to demonstrate effectiveness and efficiency.

BEYOND TREATMENT

Computers and related technology are becoming increasingly embedded in the lives of everyone, to the point that it could be argued that the world is becoming an "information society". This process seems likely to continue and people with aphasia are as much a part of this as anyone else. The final two papers in this special issue of *Aphasiology* look at ways in which computer technology may be used to supplement or augment the communicative capabilities of people with aphasia.

Van de Sandt-Koenderman looks at ways in which new technology may be used to create communication aids that may assist people with aphasia to communicate more effectively in everyday situations. Although there has been a focus on producing aids to help people who have difficulty with speech, there has been less attention paid to the needs of people with aphasia and this paper reviews the state of the art.

The paper by Egan et al. addresses the issue of the Internet and the ways in which it may be made accessible to people with aphasia. Egan et al. have developed aphasia-friendly training materials that have enabled some people with aphasia to use the Internet. This whole issue is likely to be of crucial importance in the near future, as the migration of services and information to online sources means that those without access will become increasingly disadvantaged.

FUTURE POTENTIAL

While the papers in this special issue represent real advances on the state of the art in this field, there is no reason to suppose that there are not further significant developments in store for the future. The capabilities of computer technology are continually advancing and this process is likely to continue for the foreseeable future. Also people concerned with aphasiology and with people with aphasia are likely to continue to find ever more inventive ways of exploiting that technology. An attempt to predict the future of this field in any detail would be of dubious worth; however there are some areas where the potential is clear.

New modes of treatment

Much of the work in this area has built on treatment practice in clinic, often reinforcing strategies and extending it to other settings. Developments in the field of virtual reality are now becoming available via personal computers and this will enable the creation of a more realistic context in which to address language disorders. There is a big difference between, for example, retrieving a word in response to a picture presented in a treatment context and retrieving the same word in the course of an everyday conversation. Attributing the meaning of a word is more than a merely lexical process and is likely to be affected by a range of contextual factors. Although a virtual reality language programme is not going to be a perfect analogue of everyday language use, it may well provide a kind of "half way house" which could support transfer and generalisability of clinical progress. Some of the more advanced computer-based systems for teaching foreign languages are moving in this direction.

Assessment

With the use of computer-based treatment becoming more widespread, a vast amount of data is being generated by the clients' use of these systems. Traditionally, assessment has been a distinct process whereby a standardised set of tests are undertaken at specified intervals. This mode has some disadvantages in relation to the relatively small number of questions that can be undertaken before fatigue sets in (for the client or the therapist!), and the danger that performance on assessment day may not be representative due to external factors such as mood or general wellness. The analysis of a larger set of data generated continuously may well give a more accurate account of the clients' capabilities and also be more sensitive to change.

Research and knowledge

There are two aspects to this; first, both papers in this special issue on the usefulness of computers in the treatment of aphasia identify a need for larger studies such as randomised controlled trials to provide a more solid body of evidence on which to evaluate computer-based treatment. In spite of difficulties in recruiting sufficient numbers, compounded by the variability of the condition, such studies are increasing necessary as more resources become devoted to this mode of treatment, in a healthcare context that increasingly demands high-quality evidence to justify treatments.

In many fields the availability of computer technology is enabling a increase in the pace at which knowledge is generated and there is no reason why aphasiology should not benefit in this way. The ability to rapidly analyse very large data sets and to consistently administer large volumes of tests over large numbers of people could enable significant advances to be made in areas such as enhancing and deepening the cognitive neuro-pyschological model of language processing or in exploring the relationship between memory resource allocation and linguistic performance.

Aids to living

Technology is making life easier for many of us in a variety of ways and this is already true for people with aphasia. Communication aids as described by van de Sandt-Koenderman in this issue are likely to grow in sophistication and usability. The "intelligence" that is a feature of many digital devices will enable these advances and can improve performance in aspects such as context sensitivity and improved output.

An example of how more general-purpose technical devices may help people with aphasia is the work by Wade, Petheram, and Cain (2001) which describes ways in which voice recognition technology can be used by people with aphasia as an aid to writing. Other capabilities such as text-to-speech software could assist people who can comprehend spoken messages more readily than written.

The information society

It appears to be inevitable that the importance of the Internet and associated technologies will increase. Elman (2001), and Egan et al. in this special issue of *Aphasiology*, show how this may be addressed. The potential is very exciting and goes beyond just using the Internet to access information more easily and to obtain goods and services. The Internet is a communication medium and it has the potential to ease the isolation experienced by many people with aphasia, both by facilitating contact with other people with aphasia and by enabling engagement with the many fora on the Internet. It also offers the chance for people with aphasia to express themselves and publish their experiences much more readily than was previously possible (Moss et al., in press) thus transforming them from passive consumers to active citizens.

CONCLUSION

The papers in this volume only represent a fraction of the work being done in the field of computers and aphasia. Much has been done but much remains to be done and the future is shaping up to be even more exciting than the present. Wade, Mortley, and Enderby (2003) show that people with aphasia are ready to embrace this trend and are ready to partner aphasiologists in making the possibilities a reality.

REFERENCES

Costello, J. (1977). Programmed instruction. *Journal of Speech and Hearing Disorders, 42*, 3.

Elman, R. (2001). The Internet and aphasia: Crossing the digital divide. *Aphasiology, 15*(10/11), 895–899.

Katz, R., & Nagy, V. (1982). A computerised treatment system for chronic aphasic patients. In R. H. Brookshire (Ed.), *Clinical Aphasiology Conference Proceedings*. Minneapolis: BRK Publishers.

Moss, B., Parr, S., Byng, S., & Petheram, B. (in press). "Pick me up and not a down down, up up": How are the identities of people with aphasia represented in aphasia, stroke and disability web sites? *Disability and Society*.

Wade, J., Mortley, J., & Enderby, P. (2003). Talk about IT: Views of people with aphasia and their partners on receiving remotely monitored computer-based word finding therapy. *Aphasiology*, *17*(11), 1031–1057.

Wade, J., Petheram, B., & Cain, R. (2001). Voice recognition and aphasia: Can computers understand aphasic speech? *Disability and Rehabilitation*, *23*(14), 604–613.

APHASIOLOGY, 2004, *18* (3), 193–211

Superhighway to promoting a client-therapist partnership? Using the Internet to deliver word-retrieval computer therapy, monitored remotely with minimal speech and language therapy input

Jane Mortley and Julia Wade

Speech and Language Research Unit, North Bristol NHS Trust, UK

Pam Enderby

Institute of General Practice & Primary Care, University of Sheffield, Northern General Hospital, Sheffield, UK

Background: Advances in information and communications technology have not only made independent speech and language therapy practice using a computer possible, it is now feasible to monitor this therapy from a different location ("remotely").
Aims: This paper describes an evaluation of whether therapy delivered this way is efficacious and acceptable in improving word-retrieval and efficient in terms of therapist time.
Methods & Procedures: Seven participants were recruited to a case series study, with an ABA design, where A represented a no-treatment assessment phase. All were at least 2 years post CVA and had word-finding difficulties associated with aphasia. Participants had access to therapy software on a home computer. Therapy exercises were updated remotely by a therapist from a clinic computer via the Internet. No face-to-face therapy took place.
Outcomes & Results: Outcome measures included data on software usage, pre and post-therapy language assessments, and pre and post-therapy participant interviews to explore perceived benefits and user's views. Results showed intensive use of the system, and improvement in word retrieval skills.
Conclusions: Results suggest this mode of therapy delivery is efficacious, acceptable, and gave participants a high degree of independence. Relatively little input in terms of therapist time is required. The findings are discussed in terms of implications for therapy delivery for people with aphasia.

There have been numerous studies published on the use of computers in aphasia therapy (for a review of efficacy studies see Wertz & Katz, 2004 this issue). One key finding of research to date has been that people with aphasia are able to use computers independently without a therapist present, with demonstrable benefit to the user, (Mortley, 1998;

Address correspondence to: Jane Mortley, Steps Cottage, Littleton Drew, Wiltshire SN14 7NB, UK. Email: jpmortley@btinternet.com

Jane Mortley is a director of Steps Consulting Limited, who will be commercially producing the StepByStep© software used in this paper.

The authors are extremely grateful to the seven participants and their partners for taking part in this study and to the Stroke Association for providing the funding for this research. Thanks are also due to Anthony Hughes at the Speech and Language Therapy Research Unit for his advice regarding statistics, and to Dr Sue Roulstone and Dr Brian Petheram for their comments in the preparation of this manuscript. The authors also wish to acknowledge the contribution of audience comments made at various Special Interest Group presentations, which have clarified for us some of the issues described.

DOI:10.1080/02687030344000553

Mortley, Enderby, & Petheram, 2001; Petheram, 1996; Pedersen, Vinter, & Olsen, 2001). The concept of using computers to supplement face-to-face contact with independent home-based practice is a particularly attractive one, as it has obvious resource implications (Weinrich, 1997). By their nature, computers lend themselves to repetitive drill practice and to practice alone. If a computer can be used to carry out some of the drill work previously carried out in face-to-face therapy, therapist time could be freed to spend on other tasks or with other clients. Alternatively, access to independent practice could result in increased therapy practice time without increasing therapist input. This study was conceived as an investigation of how independent home practice with a computer could be used to the benefit people with aphasia.

However, the computer is simply an alternative mode of delivering therapy and, as with any mode of therapy delivery, independent computer therapy practice continues to need close monitoring by the therapist in order to be maximally effective. This issue was raised by Pedersen et al. (2001) who suggest that their therapy, which involved the same home computer therapy programme being given to three participants, could have been made more effective by being tailored to the individual needs of participants. Monitoring and tailoring therapy in this way, however, has required face-to-face contact in the form of home visits by the therapist (Mortley et al., 2001). In the latter study, home visits were needed to be able to interpret the user's performance during unsupervised therapy tasks and refine therapy accordingly, e.g., remove exercises where performance reached ceiling or where performance demonstrated that exercises were too difficult. However, carrying out home visits is a time-consuming exercise. Gains made in terms of freeing therapist time by using the computer for independent practice are in part lost due to the need to travel. For clients living in remote rural areas, the costs of carrying out home visits may be prohibitive.

Recent advances in information and communications technology (ICT) provide a potential solution to this problem. Due to the fact that it is now possible to transfer large amounts of information via the Internet, software can be developed which will allow the therapist to assign exercises and collect exercise results on the client's computer from a physically remote location, i.e., the speech and language therapy clinic. The term "remote" is used here to mean "from a different location and without face to face contact". Studies have demonstrated that users are able to carry out practice independently. The question remains whether this practice can be monitored and adapted entirely remotely using ICT without any face-to-face contact with the therapist.

The application of computers in this way deserves investigation for three reasons. First, healthcare resources are limited. Enderby and Petheram (2002) highlight the problem that demands on speech and language therapy resources imposed by dysphagia have a negative effect on the amount of aphasia therapy available in some areas. Yet studies have suggested that a minimum of three sessions per week for not less than 5 months may be required for any positive impact on speech and language skills following stroke (Basso, Capitani, & Vignolo, 1979; Wertz et al., 1986). In the UK, the Royal College of Speech and Language Therapists recognises that many speech and language therapy services operate within a framework of insufficient resources in relation to demand (RCSLT, 1996). Any innovation that has implications for resource allocation warrants evaluation. Second, as the number of people who have access to home computers increases, the opportunity offered by computers to serve as tools for independent home practice becomes more feasible. Finally, with advances in information and communication technology, communication and information transfer between physically distant locations is becoming more efficient and reliable. Should such a method of delivering therapy prove effective, it has the potential to provide a means of modifying current SLT delivery in a way that facilitates increased therapy practice without significant increase in therapist input.

It is not only clients who are currently receiving therapy who have the potential to benefit from this technology if it proves efficacious. Evidence indicates that clients who are several years post stroke, and who have in most cases been discharged from speech and language therapy several years previously, are motivated to continue working on their communication skills and believe that they still have the potential to improve (Parr, Byng, Gilpin, & Ireland, 1997).

It is proposed that a system for delivering therapy remotely should offer the following features. Obviously, the system must be accessible and usable for people with aphasia, i.e., they must be able to carry out therapy tasks, forward results, and request new exercises independently, and therapy delivered in this manner should be acceptable to them. Second, the system must give the therapist remote access to sufficient information about the user's performance to be able to modify therapy appropriately. Third, therapy delivered in this way should be efficacious not only in treatment of language impairment (in the study described, word retrieval deficits were targeted) but also in terms of benefit to functional communication. Finally, use of the system should be efficient in terms of the ratio of therapist time required and the amount of therapy practice time obtained.

This study describes an evaluation of therapy delivered using software developed specifically with these objectives in mind. It presents an investigation of word retrieval therapy delivered remotely using a computer installed in the participant's home and connected to the therapist's computer via the Internet. The aim of the study was to evaluate the efficacy of therapy delivered in this way in terms of impact on word retrieval skills and to examine the acceptability of this mode of therapy delivery to people with aphasia. For the purpose of this report, the effects of word retrieval therapy will be examined in general terms, within the broader context of evaluating this novel mode of therapy delivery. A more detailed description and analysis of participants' impairment and therapy is contained in a separate report (Mortley, Wade, & Enderby, 2004).

METHOD

Design

A case series study was carried out using an ABACA design, in which A represented a period of assessment with no treatment and B and C represented word-finding therapy. Items for treatment were divided into Set 1 and Set 2. Following treatment to Set 1 only, (B) all items were reassessed to determine generalisation effects to Set 2, (A) after which Set 2 items were treated (C). The study was completed by a final repeat of all baseline assessments (A).

Participants

Seven participants were recruited, all with word retrieval difficulties associated with aphasia following stroke. Participants were at least 2 years post onset, discharged from therapy, and medically stable. Local therapists contacted about the study were asked to refer clients who fitted the criteria. Participants were aged between 53 and 66 years and came from a wide geographical area. Time post stroke ranged from 2 to 12 years (see Table 1 for details). Only four of the seven had previous computing experience, but all were motivated to try a computer-assisted approach to therapy.

Initial assessment included naming performance on the Object and Action Naming Battery (Druks & Masterson, 2000) and a control task, the Sentence Comprehension Assessment (Byng & Black, 1999). Assessments of word–picture matching PALPA 47 and PALPA 48 (Kay, Lesser, & Coltheart, 1992), oral reading, and patterns of response during word retrieval provided additional information to create a profile of speech and language ability for each of the seven participants (see Table 2).

TABLE 1
Participant details

	JW	BD	BH	TW	MJW	GL	GS
Age	63	53	58	63	66	63	66
Gender	M	M	M	M	F	M	M
Time post CVA	2 years	2 years	3 years	9 years	12 years	2 years	5 years
Hemiplegia	Limited use of dominant hand	No hemiplegia	Limited use of dominant hand	Limited use of dominant hand	No use of dominant hand	Hemiplegia resolved	Limited use of dominant hand
Social situation	Lives with wife	Lives with wife	Lives with wife	Lives alone	Lives with husband	Lives with wife	Lives with wife
Previous occupation	Owned village post office	Owned power tools business	Coach driver	Insurance sales	Personal assistant	Owned TV installation business	Tile fitter
Previous computer user	Yes	Yes	No	Yes	Yes	No	No

TABLE 2
Speech and language profile of participants

	JW		BD		BH		TW		MJW		GL		GS	
	raw	%	raw	%	raw	%	raw	%	raw	%	raw	%	raw	%
Object naming N = 162	46	28	68	42	87	54	70	43	70	44	56	34	48	30
Action naming N = 100	22	22	22	22	19	19	32	32	33	33	27	27	20	20
Oral reading–objects N = 81	59	72	68	84	50	61	52	64	47	58	55	68	38	46
Spoken word–picture match PALPA 47 N = 40	40	100	38	95	36.5	91	39.5	99	36	89	39	98	31.5	79
Written word–picture match PALPA 48 N = 40	35	96	38	95	36	90	40	98	30	75	39	98	25.5	64
Sentence comprehension N = 40	23	58	18	45	23	58	30	75	19	47	17	42	18	44
Summary of expressive language	Sentence structure present but marked word finding difficulties		Sentence structure present but marked word finding difficulties		Single word or 2 word utterances		2–3 word utterances, phrase level structure but few sentence level structures		Single word or 2 word utterances		Fluent speech with marked word finding difficulties and some English jargon		Single word or 2 word utterances	

Average baseline scores taken over two consecutive assessments, 6 weeks apart.

Procedures

Figure 1 summarises procedures and timescales. Language assessments, to determine the nature of word retrieval deficits and initially plan therapy, were administered face-to-face, during clinic or home visits. A home visit was then carried out to load the software onto the participant's computer (or deliver computer and software loaned) with the first set of exercises assigned for independent practice. The software was demonstrated and participants were left with instructions to use the system as much as they chose. They had access to exercise results in order to self-monitor progress over time. When ready, they forwarded results of exercises completed to the therapist via the Internet for analysis and assignment of further exercises. Having received the results, the therapist phoned the participant to discuss progress. If no results had been forwarded after 6 weeks, the therapist phoned the participant to discuss progress and agree a date for forwarding results. The therapist was available on request for face-to-face therapy sessions for any difficulties that arose.

Following analysis of results and phone discussion with the participant and carer if appropriate, the therapist selected and assigned new exercises. Exercises could be reassigned at participants' request or if usage data and results indicated that progress was likely to continue. Exercises were transferred onto the secure site on the Internet by an agreed day, ready for users to download. The cycle of transferring results and assigning new exercises continued for 3 months, after which a face-to-face assessment was carried out to determine progress on treatment and non-treatment items and whether treatment effects associated with computer-based tasks transferred to non-computer-based language tasks. Remote-based therapy then continued for a further 3 months. After completing a total of 6 months therapy, participants were asked to stop practice on exercises and were reassessed face-to-face on naming and control assessments.

Therapy was tailored to individual participants in three ways. First, the range of exercises assigned to each individual was selected from the software library of exercises (word to picture matching, semantic association, naming, reading, and spelling tasks) according to the individual's language impairment and specific goals for word retrieval therapy. Thus if written naming was a strength and a strategy of generating a phonemic cue to facilitate naming was the target of therapy, a series of exercises designed to teach this strategy was allocated to the participant. Second, once exercise selection had been made, exercises were configured as appropriate to the ability of the participant and stage of therapy, e.g., the range and complexity of target vocabulary used, and the range and type of foils used. Some participants received therapy on object names alone as opposed to object and verb names. Finally, personally relevant vocabulary was embedded into tasks in addition to the items from the naming assessment, e.g., family names or relevant place names.

Materials

Hardware.   IBM compatible PCs were used in the study. Participants used their own computer or were loaned a PC or laptop, so a range of operating systems was used (Windows 95, 98, and ME). All were supplied with a 56K modem for connection to the Internet if not already available. All used a standard mouse, speakers, and a microphone attached to the top of the monitor or clipped to the user's clothing.

Software.   StepByStep© software was developed specifically for this study and was designed with the specific needs of users with aphasia and speech and language therapists

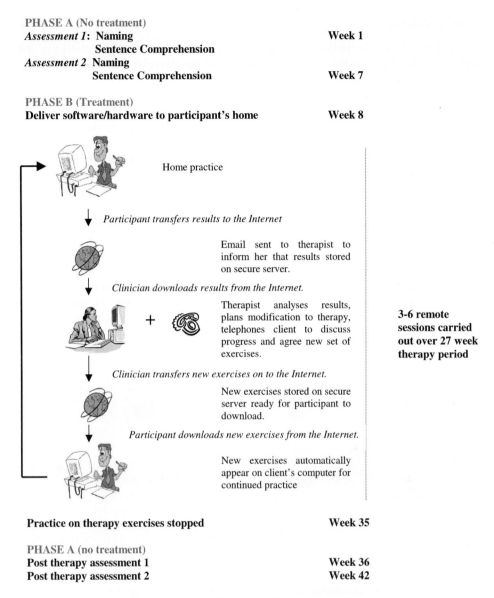

PHASE A (No treatment)
Assessment 1: **Naming**   **Week 1**
                 Sentence Comprehension
Assessment 2 **Naming**   **Week 7**
                 Sentence Comprehension

PHASE B (Treatment)
Deliver software/hardware to participant's home   **Week 8**

Home practice

Participant transfers results to the Internet

Email sent to therapist to inform her that results stored on secure server.

Clinician downloads results from the Internet.

Therapist analyses results, plans modification to therapy, telephones client to discuss progress and agree new set of exercises.

3-6 remote sessions carried out over 27 week therapy period

Clinician transfers new exercises on to the Internet.

New exercises stored on secure server ready for participant to download.

Participant downloads new exercises from the Internet.

New exercises automatically appear on client's computer for continued practice

Practice on therapy exercises stopped   **Week 35**

PHASE A (no treatment)
Post therapy assessment 1   **Week 36**
Post therapy assessment 2   **Week 42**

Figure 1. Overview of procedures for assessment and therapy.

in mind. In order to enable remote delivery and monitoring of therapy, it incorporated not only a user interface with therapy software, but also an Internet update facility to enable transfer of data to and from the user, and a therapist interface to enable remote monitoring of therapy (see Figure 1). Some of the features of the therapist interface were developed during the course of the study, as it became apparent that processes could be automated to benefit the therapist in terms of time required for monitoring therapy. All components of the user interface were in place at the outset.

User interface

The user interface was designed so that the user could not only access and carry out exercises independently, but also transfer results to the therapist and download newly assigned exercises unaided.

Access to and nature of therapy exercises.   The software system was accessed via an icon on the desk-top. Exercises were assigned a name meaningful to the client (e.g., "Similar pictures" for a semantic association task). A maximum of 15 exercises could be assigned at any one time. The wide range of therapy tasks reproduced by the software included spoken and written word–picture matching tasks, semantic association, naming, reading, and spelling tasks (Figure 2). Tasks used photographs, sound, and text as appropriate. Responses required varied according to task, e.g., multiple choice selection in word to picture matching; spoken production for recording by the software in naming; keyboard entry for spelling. (For more details on therapy see Mortley et al., 2004).

Feedback during therapy tasks.   The software responded to user difficulties by making tasks easier when errors were made and by enabling the user to request cues as required. Feedback depended on the type of exercise. For example in naming tasks (Figure 2iv), the user was able to request any one from a hierarchy of cues ranging from

i) Semantic association task

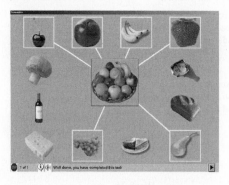

ii) Spelling task

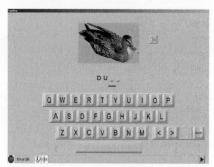

iii) Written word to picture matching task

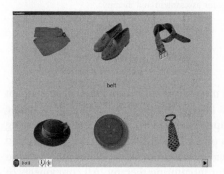

iv) Naming task

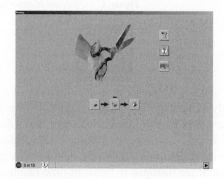

Figure 2.   Sample exercises from StepByStep©.

the initial letter, initial sound, or initial syllable to the whole word for repetition. In word–picture matching tasks, every word or picture displayed had a digitised recording of its spoken name available for playback so that this additional auditory cue could be heard on request. If an incorrect item was chosen, the picture selection was reduced to three items, and if another incorrect response was made the target was revealed. In writing tasks, the number of letters from which to choose was reduced if the user chose incorrectly. In summary, the software was designed to respond constructively to user difficulties, but also allow the user some choice in the nature of support she or he could request.

Feedback on performance.   The user determined when they wanted to forward results for analysis by the therapist. Progress could be reviewed at any time, and feedback included the number of correct responses per exercise and number of attempts at each exercise and a graphical analysis of progress on one exercise over time. During production tasks (naming or repetition) users were able to record multiple attempts at production for playback and self-monitoring. When satisfied with the quality of production they could save their recording for the therapist to listen to when accessing results.

Transfer of data via the Internet.   It was assumed that users might have no prior knowledge of computers or the Internet. Transfer of data from and to the user's computer was therefore designed to be a single fully automated procedure. The user switched to the Update screen and clicked on a telephone icon. This activated the transfer of results data to the secure server on the Internet. A series of traffic-light icons changing from red to green as each step in the process was successfully completed, provided the user with visual feedback of the process. The steps automated in this way are summarised in Figure 3. Steps 1–3 were relevant for exporting results. Following phone discussion and analysis of results, the therapist assigned exercises for the user to collect from the server. Exercises were collected by the user repeating the automated Update procedure, but at this stage of data transfer, steps 4–5 were relevant.

Therapist interface

This was designed with the aim of reducing time taken to monitor and modify therapy remotely to a minimum, by automating as many processes as possible. The therapist needed to be able to monitor several different clients from the clinic computer. A large library of exercises was needed, from which exercises appropriate to the individual could quickly and efficiently be assigned to users. Results data needed to be analysed easily and efficiently, and transfer of data via the Internet needed to be efficient and reliable.

User management.   The therapist managed each client by accessing a dropdown menu and selecting the relevant client under the heading ''patient''. From here the

---

1. Retrieve latest results from the computer and compress them in preparation for sending.
2. Connect to the safe server on the Internet using dial-up networking.
3. Transfer results to safe server.
4. Establish whether any new exercises were awaiting collection and download them into the appropriate directory with appropriate speech and sound files attached.
5. Update the exercise screen with new exercises and display for user.

Figure 3.   Steps automated in data transfer.

therapist was able to carry out all tasks relevant to that client, importing and exporting data, analysing results, and assigning exercises as appropriate.

Assigning exercises from the library.   Exercises were tailored to individual needs by adjusting a range of different parameters, e.g., number of foils displayed, whether foils were written, pictured, or both, and the psycholinguistic variables of the target and foils in terms of imageability, frequency, age of acquisition. In order to specify parameters and create the desired exercise easily, an exercise design interface was developed. Once specified, the therapist could preview an exercise before assigning it. New exercises were designed in response to individual needs, with the result that the exercise library was much larger and more comprehensive by the time the study was completed.

Results monitoring and data transfer.   Computer usage data, including what exercises were carried out and what errors were made, were captured automatically by the software. During the study, the software was further refined to enable the automatic generation of a report for ease of analysis and to save therapist time, and the processes involved in retrieving results from the Internet and transferring them to the correct directory on the clinician's computer were fully automated. Similarly, once the therapist had assigned new exercises to a client, all associated files (e.g., picture and sound files) were identified and transferred automatically.

Outcome measures

A range of outcome measures was used to investigate use of the system by participants and evaluate the efficacy of therapy delivered. Usage data captured automatically by the software investigated individual patterns of use, and non-computer-administered language assessments conducted before and after therapy investigated efficacy of therapy in terms of benefit to word retrieval. Semi-structured interviews sought to investigate participants' views on acceptability of this mode of therapy delivery as well as explore perceived benefits.

Usage data.   The automatic data capture facility of the software enabled recording of a range of aspects of usage for analysis. These are summarised in Figure 4.

Language assessments.   Baseline assessments were carried out on the naming battery items targeted in therapy (Druks & Masterson, 2000) and a sentence-processing assessment (Byng & Black, 1999), a control task not expected to show change from therapy.

- Total hours practice over 27 week period
- Average practice time per month, per week, per session
- Number of active weeks, days
- Total no of exercises assigned, carried out
- Average number of attempts per exercise
- Average number of exercises per week
- Average number of exercises per session
- No. of correct responses on each exercise
- No. of cues requested on each exercise

Figure 4.   Summary of usage data captured by the software.

Baseline measures were repeated a minimum of 6 weeks apart in order to determine their stability. Post-therapy measures were also taken twice, one within 1 week of finishing therapy and one a minimum of 6 weeks after withdrawal of therapy, to measure maintenance. An additional assessment of all the naming battery items was carried out following treatment to Set 1 in order to determine whether there was evidence of generalisation to non-treatment items, Set 2. The black and white line drawings of the naming battery determined whether improvements on naming the computer stimuli (photographs) generalised to naming other stimuli.

Interviews.   Semi-structured interviews were carried out by a therapist not involved in giving therapy with six of the seven participants and (where applicable) with their carers in order to explore views on acceptability of this mode of therapy delivery. Interview data is reported in more detail elsewhere (Wade, Mortley, & Enderby, 2003). A brief summary of evidence for perceived benefit and views on acceptability is presented here.

RESULTS

Usage data

The usage data for the seven participants is reported in Table 3. In analysing results, it should be borne in mind that figures represent the time spent actively engaged in performing exercises, i.e., excluding time spent switching on the computer, reviewing results, updating exercises, swapping or pausing between exercises, or indeed any periods when the software was left on but inactive.

All seven participants continued to use the software throughout the 27-week therapy period. All periods of inactivity recorded were accounted for by participants' holiday and/ or periods when technical difficulties disrupted use of the software (e.g., TW and BH; see below). Following these breaks, use recommenced with a similar intensity to before, so there was no reduction in intensity of use over the 27 weeks. Some parameters of use showed a far greater range across the group than others. The group mean for the total number of hours' practice was 74 hours 20 minutes, (range = 46 h 48 to 92 h 43) and the group mean for the number of hours' practice per month was 12 hours 23 minutes (range = 7 h 48 to 15 h 27). The group mean for the average number of hours' practice per week was 2 hours 45 minutes (range = 1 h 43 to 3 h 46). The group mean for the total number of exercises assigned was 39, (range = 16–70 exercises) and the group mean for the average number of attempts per exercise was 14 (range = 6–44). The range on these latter two parameters was particularly broad. This reflects the fact that therapy was monitored by the therapist and tailored to the preferences expressed by individuals, e.g., some participants preferred to continue working on exercises until performance was close to 100%.

Once the therapist interface of the software had been refined to automate as many processes as possible, remote sessions lasted on average 2 hours each. This time included the therapist downloading results, phoning the participant to discuss progress, agreeing what exercises to assign, designing these, and transferring them to the secure server. The length of remote sessions varied according to the length of the phone conversation and the need to create any exercises specific to the individual that were not stored in the library. The only therapy contact with the therapist during the 6-month period was the phone conversations during remote sessions. No participants requested additional face-to-face therapy via home visits. Home visits were used solely to solve technical difficulties

TABLE 3
Usage data for seven participants

	JW	BD	BH	TW	MJW	GL	GS	Group Average
Total time spent	88 h 9 min	88 h 48 min	57 h 21 min	46 h 48 min	92 h 43 min	73 h 38 min	73 h 20 min	74 h 23 min
Average time per month	14 h 41 min	14 h 48 min	9 h 30 min	7 h 48 min	15 h 27 min	12 h 16 min	12 h 20 min	12 h 23 min
Average time per week	3 h 15 min	3 h 17 min	2 h 7 min	1 h 43 min	3 h 26 min	3 h 17 min	2 h 43 min	2 h 45 min
Average time per session	52 min	1 hr 11 min	47 min	38 min	37 min	46 min	48 min	48 min
No. of active weeks (max = 27)	22	24	14	14	25	22	19	20
No. of active days (max = 184)	101	79	68	71	147	88	96	78
Total number of exercises assigned	70	53	44	54	50	55	16	39
Average no. of attempts per exercise	9	13	9	6	18	11	44	14
Average no. of exercises per week	26	27	20	21	34	22	32	22
Average no. of exercises per session	6	9	6	4	6	6	7	5

or to carry out interim language assessments. All participants demonstrated the ability to carry out therapy tasks, forward results, and download new exercises independently of carers.

Aside from pre-scheduled assessment visits, three participants requested additional home visits during the 6-month therapy period. JW and BH had technical difficulties caused by the modem. A home visit to replace the modem solved the problem (two home visits each). TW mistakenly erased the contents of his hard drive. The hard drive was collected, reconfigured, the software reloaded, and the PC returned (two home visits). The number of remote therapy sessions per participant over the 27-week period ranged from three to six. GS required fewer remote sessions because he chose to work on each exercise for longer, attempting each 44 times compared to the group mean of 14.

Language data

Table 4 summarises results of naming assessments and sentence comprehension assessment (control task) pre- and post-therapy. Baseline performance on object and action naming assessments showed stable performance prior to the start of therapy. The mean of the two pre-therapy scores was therefore taken as a baseline, against which to compare post therapy results. Table 5 shows the results of the interim language assessment following treatment (B) to Set 1 only.

Naming.   Results for the 162-item object naming assessment showed a significant improvement in the ability to retrieve object names for each of the seven participants (JW: $z = 13.28, p < .001$; BD: $z = 8.2, p < .001$; BH: $z = 7.01, p < .001$; TW: $z = 5.00, p < .001$; MJW: $z = 3.80, p < .001$; GL: $z = 5.92, p < .001$, GS: $z = 5.5, p < .001$). Results for the 100-item action naming assessment showed a significant improvement in the ability to retrieve action names for six of the seven participants (JW: $z = 9.44, p < .001$; BD: $z = 5.46, p < .001$; BH: $z = 8.34, p < .001$; TW: $z = 4.12, p < .001$; MJW: $z = 3.85, p < .001$; GL: $z = 3.89, p < .001$). Although improvement was observed for TW at the first post-therapy assessment, it did not reach significance until the time of the second, maintenance assessment. Verbs were not targeted in therapy for GS, so no improvement in action naming was anticipated for him.

Results of the interim object naming assessments, administered after set 1 had been treated (Table 5) showed generalisation to untreated items (Set 2) for three of the seven participants JW: 28–43% ($z = 2.36, p < .009$); BD: 39–56% ($z = 2.48, p < .006$); BH: 54.5–72%, ($z = 2.71, p < .003$). Generalisation to untreated items for TW, MJW, GL, and GS did not take place.

Control assessment.   Results for the 40-item sentence comprehension assessment indicated that no significant change in performance had taken place for any of the participants. The lack of change on this control assessment, combined with the stable baseline scores on naming, suggest that improvements in naming ability are unlikely to be the result of spontaneous recovery.

Interview data

Acceptability.   All six participants interviewed perceived remotely monitored computer therapy as a positive experience. Although no interview was carried out with GS, he and his carer indicated that he had enjoyed the therapy so much that he was

TABLE 4

Language assessment results

	JW		BD		BH		TW		MJW		GL		GS	
	raw	%	raw	%	raw	%	raw	%	raw	%	raw	%	raw	%
Object naming (n = 162)														
pre 1	42	26	58	36	84	52	71	44	64	40	51	31	42	26
pre 2	49	30	78	48	89	55	68	42	76	47	60	37	53	33
average pre score	46	28	68	42	87	54	70	43	70	44	56	34	48	30
post 1	119	73	117	72	132	81	104	64	109	67	81	50	87	54
post 2	131	81	125	77	133	82	107	66	99	61	100	62	89	55
Action naming (n = 100)														
pre 1	22	22	17	17	20	20	30	30	33	33	25	25	20	20
pre 2	21	21	26	26	18	18	33	33	33	33	29	29	20	20
average pre score	22	22	22	22	19	19	32	32	33	33	27	27	20	20
post 1	61	61	50	50	67	67	43	43	54	54	48	48	29	29
post 2	72	72	53	53	65	65	56	56	56	56	48	48	27	27
Sentence comprehension (control) (N = 40)														
pre 1	22	55	16	40	22	55	28	70	19	48	17	43	19	48
pre 2	24	60	20	50	24	60	32	80	18	45	16	40	16	40
average pre score	23	58	18	45	23	58	30	75	19	47	17	44	18	44
post	22	55	17	43	20	50	33	83	21	53	15	38	17	43

TABLE 5
Pre-therapy and interim scores for naming nouns

	JW		BD		BH		TW		MW		GL		GS	
	raw	%	raw	%	raw	%	raw	%	raw	%	raw	%	raw	%
Set 1 Average baseline	23	28	36.5	45	42.5	52	38	47	36	44	32	39	26.5	33
Set 1 Interim (treated)	61	75	64	79	67	83	61	75	51	63	57	70	41	51
Set 2 Average baseline	22.5	28	31.5	39	44	54	31.5	39	34	42	23.5	29	21	26
Set 2 Interim (untreated)	35	43	45	56	58	72	38	47	36	44	31	38	21	26

distressed to see it end. This model of therapy delivery was particularly valued because it allowed the user to determine timing and intensity of practice, and participants were able to self-monitor their performance. The regular phone contact with the therapist was highlighted as important in maintaining motivation. All participants valued the face-to-face contact with the therapist to carry out assessments.

Perceived benefits.   All interviewees reported a perceived improvement in their ability to name items targeted in therapy (as confirmed in language data) and all reported a perceived change in functional communication (see Figure 5 for a list of evidence cited). Four of the six interviewees (JW, BD, BH, and GL) were able to report concrete examples of new activities undertaken as a result of increased confidence following therapy (see Figure 5 for a list of examples cited). For JW and GL, the regular phone discussions with the therapist had generalised to spontaneous independent use of the phone.

DISCUSSION

This study set out to evaluate whether the software developed would enable independent practice by people with aphasia, which could be monitored and adapted remotely via the Internet by a speech and language therapist without face-to-face contact, and to investigate the impact of therapy on word finding. It was argued that a system for delivering therapy remotely should be accessible, usable, and acceptable to people with aphasia, and should give the therapist remote access to sufficient information about the user's performance to be able to modify therapy appropriately. Therapy delivered in this way should be efficacious in treatment of both language impairment (in this case, word retrieval) and functional communication. Finally, use of the system should be efficient in terms of the ratio of therapist time required to the amount of therapy practice time obtained. Each of these will be discussed, before turning to a more general consideration of issues raised by the study.

All participants demonstrated the ability and the motivation to use the software independently, with neither speech and language therapist nor carer present. The group

Participant	Reported evidence of benefits to functional communication	Reported new activities and behaviours
JW	• Initiating communication with strangers • Increased participation in group conversations • Using phone • Shopping without a list • Writing letters	• Enrolled on computer course • Return to driving • Increased walking
BD	• Taking time to find words • Initiating conversation with neighbours • Shopping alone • Answering phone • Discussing current affairs	• Preparing meals unaided • Doing car maintenance using manual • Assisting friend to rewire house • Using Internet as info source
BH	• Producing more phrases • Increased participation in family conversations • Needing fewer repetitions • Using family names • Buying petrol alone	• Decorating house • Laughing at jokes on TV/in conversations
TW	• Producing more phrases • Finding words more easily • Reading the newspaper	
MJW	• Finding words targeted in therapy more easily • Asserting self more to ensure message is understood • Increased participation in communication	
GL	• More aware of errors and better able to correct • Strangers don't always notice aphasia • Using phone • Using family names • Attempting to write	• Using Internet • Improved confidence with computers • Improved moods

Figure 5. Reported benefits to functional communication and examples of new activities or behaviours noted since start of therapy.

mean showed that participants spent an average of 2 hours 45 minutes per week and 12 hours 23 minutes per month on therapy tasks, an impressive outcome, given that they determined frequency of use for themselves. The consistent use of the software by all in the group throughout the therapy period is indicative of the degree of continued motivation maintained by all participants. All reported that this mode of therapy delivery was acceptable and having control over intensity and duration of any practice was particularly valued. The wide range of therapy tasks that could be presented on the software may also have been a factor in maintaining motivation.

The transfer of data via the Internet also proved to be within the capacity of all participants, even those with moderate–severe aphasia. Although participants were self-selecting in this study, in that they were all keen to try a computer-assisted approach to therapy, three of them had little or no prior experience of using computers. In this light, the degree of independence demonstrated in carrying out therapy tasks and transferring results is very encouraging.

However, of far greater significance than participants' ability to use the system, is the evidence provided by language assessments that use of the therapy software benefited language skills for all of them. Given the fact that all therapy in this study was delivered via the computer, the only face-to-face contact being to carry out assessments or solve technical difficulties, the results of the language assessments, which showed a significant improvement in naming ability for all seven participants, are encouraging. This clearly demonstrates the transfer of learning from the computer-administered therapy tasks to non-computer-based picture-naming assessments. This improvement was shown on a large number of items targeted in therapy (i.e., 262 items for six participants and 162 items for one participant), and generalisation to non-treatment items was found for three participants.

Moreover, the improvement was not restricted to performance on language assessments, as all participants reported increased confidence and participation in communication as a result of therapy. Four participants and their carers were able to give specific examples of how communication had changed over the therapy period. Examples such as being more aware and better able to correct errors, not relying on their partner to "fill in words", shopping independently without needing words written down, using the phone for the first time, and using family names for the first time, were felt to be evidence for some degree of functional carryover. As regards the remaining three participants, although they reported that they felt communication had improved, for example in being able to find words more easily, communicating more, or reading more, these claims could not be backed up by specific examples, and so provide less convincing evidence of functional carryover.

In-depth interviews enabled individual responses to this mode of therapy delivery to be explored in greater detail, in addition to exploring evidence of functional benefit. This is one of the strengths of this methodology, making it particularly appropriate for investigating a novel form of therapy delivery (Damico, Simmons-Mackie, Oelshlaeger, Elman, & Armstrong, 1999; Pope, Ziebland, & Mays, 2000). The nature of this evidence must nevertheless be borne in mind in interpretation, i.e., evidence of functional benefit is based on participant and carer report rather than independent report or external measurement tool. Recent studies evaluating word retrieval have investigated carryover into everyday communication by sampling spontaneous speech before and after therapy (Hickin, Best, Herbert, Howard, & Osborne, 2001). The analysis of spontaneous speech sampled before and after therapy in this study would have shed further light on the issue of functional carryover.

The question remains as to the relative efficiency of this mode of delivering therapy. Comparison of the time taken to carry out a remote therapy session (average 2 hours a month), with the amount of therapy practice time that participants carried out in response to a remote session (average 12 hours 23 minutes per month), suggests that this is, indeed, a highly efficient way of delivering word retrieval therapy. The average practice time undertaken by this group per week (2 hours 45 minutes) is comparable to the intensity recommended by the RCSLT for people with aphasia of three sessions per week (RCSLT, 1996). The proportion of therapy time to therapist time is favourable compared to conventional face-to-face contact. It also compares favourably to computer therapy practice, which is carried out at home but requires home visits by the speech and language therapist to monitor progress and modify accordingly. Three key features of the software design led to substantial time savings for the therapist: first, the generation of a summary of results for analysis and planning of therapy; second, the facility for results to be transferred without both therapist and participant being present simultaneously; finally, the large and easily accessed exercise library. This was only made possible as a result of the software being developed with the specific needs of both users with aphasia and therapists in mind. It begs the question of what further processes can be automated to the benefit of both users and therapists. Finally, it should be noted that the relative efficiency of this mode of therapy delivery will also depend on the ready availability of technical support to sort out difficulties with software or hardware.

It is interesting to note that this improvement took place without any face-to-face therapy. This study has demonstrated that word retrieval therapy does not necessarily need to be administered by a therapist, particularly in the cases such as JW, BD, and BH where generalisation to untreated items occurred and concrete examples of changes in functional communication were provided during the interviews. The results call for a reappraisal of the role of the therapist in such cases. If a computer can be used to administer tasks focusing specifically on language impairment, the therapist could focus more on activities that continue to require therapist input, for example, analysis of assessment results and planning therapy, the establishment of positive conversational strategies between the person with aphasia and their partner, or counselling. It could be argued that if TW, MJW, GL, and GS had received face-to-face therapy, then the impact of therapy may have been greater. As software applications become more sophisticated, therapists will no doubt be challenged to examine their assumptions about what parts of the therapy process can be automated. Appropriate tasks include some aspects of assessment. Further research is clearly needed to determine whether this is feasible.

Another interesting finding of the study was that this mode of therapy delivery shifted the locus of control towards the client. Although the therapist continued to assign therapy tasks, this was done very much in consultation with participants and in response to participant feedback, e.g., participants might request an exercise be left to practise longer. This consultation process came about in part because the therapist was not present to witness tasks being performed. Although information on performance could be gleaned from the results' report, the therapist was also reliant on participant feedback during monthly phone calls. The result was a process of joint negotiation by which the next set of therapy exercises was agreed. Moreover, in carrying out exercises, participants determined when, for how long, and how they carried out therapy tasks. Individual variations that the system allowed included deciding when to request a model, when to request a cue, and how many attempts to make at producing a target item before saving the recording for the therapist to monitor. The usage data demonstrated a wide range of approaches taken by individuals in their pattern of practice. Clearly further research is needed to investigate whether this variation is linked to learning style and personality, or to the nature of the language impairment, or other unknown factors. The software represents a new tool with which to analyse the ways in which people with aphasia differ in their approach to learning or therapy practice. Investigating individual preferences in therapy styles may shed light on what is appropriate for different individuals.

Finally, this study raises the question of what is the appropriate timing for intervention using remotely delivered computer therapy. All participants reported here were at least 2 years post onset. The unmet needs in terms of therapy provision of people living with long-term aphasia have never been clearly documented and quantified, although evidence suggests that there is a perceived need for speech and language therapy several years post onset (Parr et al., 1997). This mode of therapy delivery may offer the potential to meet some of this need at relatively little cost.

CONCLUSION

This study has demonstrated that remotely delivered computer therapy was efficacious when delivered to the seven participants in this study in the context of a research study. The next challenge will be to determine whether it is an effective and efficient mode of service delivery when used in service context and if so for whom.

REFERENCES

Basso, A., Capitani, E., & Vignolo, L. A. (1979). Influence of rehabilitation in language skills in aphasic patients: A controlled study. *Archives of Neurology, 36*, 190–196.

Byng, S., & Black, M. (1999). *The Reversible Sentences Comprehension Test.* Bicester, UK: Winslow Press Ltd.

Damico, J., Simmons-Mackie, N., Oelshlaeger, M., Elman, R., & Armstrong, A. (1999). Qualitative methods in aphasia research: Basic issues. *Aphasiology, 13*, 9–11, 651–665.

Druks, J., & Masterson, J. (2000). *An object and action naming battery.* Hove, UK: Psychology Press.

Enderby, P., & Petheram, B. (2002). Has aphasia therapy been swallowed up? *Clinical Rehabilitation, 16*(6), 604–608.

Hickin, J., Best, W., Herbert, R., Howard, D., & Osborne, F. (2001). Treatment of word retrieval in aphasia: Generalisation to conversational speech. *International Journal of Language and Communication Disorders, 36*(Suppl), 13–18.

Kay, J., Lesser, R., & Coltheart, M. (1992). *Psycholinguistic Assessment of Language Processing in Aphasia (PALPA).* Hove, UK: Lawrence Erlbaum Associates Ltd.

Mortley, J. (1998). *Evaluating the efficacy of targeted intensive therapy facilitated by computer administered to dysphasic individuals.* PhD thesis, University of Exeter, UK.

Mortley, J., Enderby, P., & Petheram, P. (2001). Using a computer to improve functional writing in a patient with severe dysgraphia. *Aphasiology, 15*(5) 443–461.

Mortley, J., Wade, J., & Enderby, P. M. (2004). *The impact of remotely monitored word retrieval computer therapy*: A case series study. Manuscript submitted for publication.

Parr, S., Byng, S., Gilpin, S., & Ireland, C. (1997). *Talking about aphasia: Living with loss of language after stroke.* Buckingham, UK: Open University Press.

Pedersen, P. M., Vinter, K., & Olsen, T. S. (2001). Improvement of oral naming by unsupervised computerised rehabilitation. *Aphasiology, 15*, 151–169.

Petheram, B. (1996). Exploring the home-based use of microcomputers in aphasia therapy. *Aphasiology, 10*(3), 267–82.

Pope, C., Ziebland, S., & Mays, N. (2000). Analysing qualitative data. *British Medical Journal, 320*, 114–116.

Royal College of Speech and Language Therapists (1996). *Communicating Quality 2, Professional standards for speech and language therapists* (p. 272). London: Royal College of Speech and Language Therapists.

StepByStep© (2003). [Software] Steps Consulting Limited, Steps Cottage, Littleton Drew, Wiltshire SN14 7NB, UK. www.stepstherapy.co.uk

Wade, J., Mortley, J., & Enderby, P. M. (2003). Talk about IT: Views of people with aphasia and their partners on receiving remotely monitored computer-based word finding therapy. *Aphasiology, 17*, 1031–1056.

Weinrich, M. (1997). Computer rehabilitation in aphasia. *Clinical Neuroscience, 4*, 103–107.

Wertz, R. T., & Katz, R. (2004). Outcomes of computer-provided treatment for aphasia. *Aphasiology, 18*(3), 229–244.

Wertz, R. T., Weiss, D. G., Aten, J., Brookshire, R. H., Garcia-Bunuel, L., Holland, A. et al. (1986). Comparison of clinic, home and deferred language treatment for aphasia: Veterans Administration Cooperative Study. *Archives of Neurology, 43*, 653–658.

APHASIOLOGY, 2004, *18* (3), 213–222

Cues on request: The efficacy of Multicue, a computer program for wordfinding therapy

Suzanne J. C. Doesborgh

Erasmus MC, Rotterdam, The Netherlands

Mieke W. M. E. van de Sandt-Koenderman

*Rijndam Rehabilitation Centre/Rotterdam Aphasia Foundation, Rotterdam,
The Netherlands*

Diederik W. J. Dippel, Frans van Harskamp, Peter J. Koudstaal,
and Evy G. Visch-Brink

Erasmus MC, Rotterdam, The Netherlands

Background: Semantic and word form cues have been shown to have long-term effects on naming in aphasia. Multicue is a computer program that offers a variety of cues for improving word finding. It stimulates the users' independence by encouraging them to discover themselves which cues are most helpful.

Aims: We investigated the effects of Multicue on naming and verbal communication.

Methods & Procedures: A total of 18 individuals with aphasia caused by stroke, who had completed intensive impairment-oriented treatment, were randomised to 10–11 hours of Multicue ($n = 8$) or no treatment ($n = 10$).

Outcomes & Results: Only the Multicue group improved on the Boston Naming Test. However, mean improvement did not differ significantly between the treated and untreated groups, neither for the BNT (95% CI: -4.5 to 26.1), nor for the ANELT-A (95% CI: -2.4 to 9.4).

Conclusions: In the chronic phase of aphasia, following impairment-oriented treatment, Multicue may have a beneficial effect on word finding in picture naming, but not on verbal communication. The effect of Multicue may be the result either of self-cueing or of improved access. The lack of generalisation to verbal communication is discussed.

Address correspondence to: Mieke W. M. E. van de Sandt-Koenderman, Rijndam Rehabilitation Centre/ Rotterdam Aphasia Foundation, Westersingel 300, 3015 LJ Rotterdam, The Netherlands.
Email: m.sandt@rijndam.nl

The study is supported by the Netherlands Organisation for Scientific Research. We are very grateful to the persons with aphasia for their willing participation. We also thank their speech and language therapists from the following clinical centres: *Hospital:* Erasmus MC (Rotterdam). *Rehabilitation centres:* Beatrixoord (Gronin-gen), Kastanjehof (Apeldoorn), Het Roessingh (Enschede). *Rehabilitation departments of nursing homes:* Antonius IJsselmonde, Elf Ranken, Schiehoven-Wilgenplas, Rheuma (all connected to Rotterdam Aphasia Foundation), Rustoord (Sassenheim), De Plantage (Brielle), Zonnekamp (Steenwijk), Hartkamp (Raalte). *Private practices:* Stichting Afasietherapie Amsterdam, Praktijk voor Logopedie Soest, Logopediepraktijk van Gol (Harderwijk), Logopediepraktijk Halk-Meyer (Rhoon), Afasiecentrum Rotterdam e.o. (Capelle a/d IJssel).

Many thanks to M. van Rijn for her assistance with testing and collecting data.

In this study we investigated the efficacy of Multicue (Van de Sandt-Koenderman, & Visch-Brink, 1993; Van Mourik & Van de Sandt-Koenderman, 1992), a computer therapy for improving word finding. Multicue uses a variety of cueing techniques to promote self-cueing strategies in aphasia. Cueing is a common technique in word finding treatment. When a person with aphasia experiences difficulties in finding a word, a semantic, phonological, or orthographic cue may provide additional information and help to activate the target word above threshold (Avila, Lambon Ralph, Parcet, Geffner, & Gonzalez-Darder, 2001).

Howard and Orchard-Lisle (1984) distinguished three ways in which cueing may have an effect: (1) cues may have a direct effect (a "prompting" effect), (2) cues may have an effect at a later point in time (a "facilitation" effect), or (3) cues may have a permanent effect, not only on the target word, but also on other words (a "therapeutic" effect). To achieve a therapeutic effect cues should be repeatedly applied. They are often presented in a hierarchical format from least informative to most informative, e.g., first phoneme, first syllable, whole word for repetition (e.g., Hickin, Best, Herbert, Howard, & Osborne, 2002a; Hillis, 1989).

EFFICACY OF CUEING TREATMENTS

Previous studies have shown positive effects of cueing treatments on naming. In many single and multiple case studies the long-term effect of semantic cueing treatment on naming was established, not only on trained but also on untrained items (Coelho, McHugh, & Boyle, 2000; Drew & Thompson, 1999; Wambaugh et al., 2001). The positive effects of phonological techniques have also been noted (Hickin et al., 2002a). In a review of word finding therapy, Nickels (2002) concludes that semantic and phonological techniques are effective, and she suggests that a combination of both may prove to be most effective.

As orthographic cues may assist in retrieving the phonological word form, these cues are often used in treatment. The effect of treatment based on orthographic cues is reported to be equally effective as (Hickin et al., 2002a) or more effective than (Basso, Marangolo, Piras, & Galluzzi, 2001) treatment based on phonological cues. A well-known orthographic approach involves reteaching the link between phonology and orthography to individuals with aphasia who have better written than spoken naming. Once grapheme–phoneme conversion is relearned, the person with aphasia can use the available orthographic information to generate his or her own phonological cues. This strategy can be applied to any word, and therefore generalisation to untrained words is expected (Nickels, 2002).

The effect of cueing treatments on verbal communication is unknown. It is often implicitly assumed that improved performance on a naming task brings about improved verbal communication, but this is hardly supported by research. Of over 50 studies investigating the efficacy of impairment-oriented word finding treatment, only a handful explicitly looked at generalisation to spontaneous speech, with contradictory results (Boyle & Coelho, 1995; Doesborgh, van de Sandt-Koenderman, Dippel, van Harskamp, Koudstaal, & Visch-Brink, 2004; Franklin, Buerk, & Howard, 2002; Hickin, Herbert, Best, Howard, & Osborne, 2002b; McNeil et al., 1997).

Although much is known about the efficacy of different cueing techniques on naming, it is not fully understood which cues are suitable for which individuals. There is no simple one-to-one relationship between the loci of impairment and the cues that will facilitate word finding: semantic techniques can improve naming for individuals with good semantic processing (Nickels & Best, 1996) and phonological tasks can improve naming for individuals with semantic impairments (Nickels, 2002; Raymer, Thompson, Jacobs, & Le Grand, 1993). Multicue's approach to tailoring therapy to the individual is to supply persons with aphasia with a range of different cues and encourage them to discover for themselves which cues they find most suitable (i.e., "discovery-based learning").

MULTICUE

The basic idea in Multicue is to let the person with aphasia experience the effect of several cues on his or her word finding problems. In a naming task, the user has to find out which cues are most helpful and to discover which information he or she may already have available. In contrast with many cueing therapies, there is no fixed, pre-conceived cueing hierarchy; instead, the user is free to select any cue. By experiencing the success of different cues, users gain insight into which cues are most suitable to complete their partial knowledge of the word. This may enable them to develop self-cueing strategies by internalising the relevant parts of the cueing system.

Computers have been used with success for aphasia therapy in general (Aftonomos, Appelbaum, & Steele, 1999; Stachowiak, 1993) and also specifically for word finding therapy (Bruce & Howard, 1987; Colby, Christinaz, Parkinson, Graham, & Karpf, 1981; Deloche et al., 1992; Fink, Brecher, Schwartz, & Robey, 2002; Van Mourik et al., 1992). Several studies comparing computer therapy to therapist-delivered therapy found comparable effects (Kinsey, 1990; Van de Sandt-Koenderman et al., 1993). An important advantage of computer programs is that they allow the user to work independently and to decide how much time to spend on a particular word without being judged by the therapist. Multicue thus enables the aphasic user to control his or her own word finding process.

In a previous study, three of four participants with chronic aphasia improved their oral naming of untrained items by 10–20% after treatment with Multicue for 3–6 weeks, whereas none of the participants showed better results after the paper-and-pencil version of the same therapy, provided by a clinician (Van Mourik et al., 1992).

In this study, we have investigated clinically relevant effects of Multicue in a group of persons with naming disorders. Their gains on naming and everyday language were contrasted with the gains of an untreated control group. As Multicue takes a strategic approach, we neither aimed at nor expected an improvement that was confined to the items used in therapy; the learned strategies were supposed to be independent of the particular words used in therapy and consequently should have an effect on untrained words and modalities as well. We therefore hypothesised that training with Multicue, a program with written cues and written feedback, would result in improved oral naming of untrained items, with generalisation to verbal communication.

METHOD

Participants

Persons with aphasia after stroke who had completed intensive impairment-oriented (semantic or phonological) therapy were asked to participate in this study. They were included in the study if they met the following inclusion criteria: age 20–86, native Dutch speaker, no developmental dyslexia or illiteracy, no global aphasia or rest-aphasia, at least 11 months post stroke onset, and a moderate/severe naming deficit (Boston Naming Test < 120 out of 180, Dutch scoring system, Van Loon-Vervoorn, Stumpel, & De Vries,

1995, see Appendix A). Informed consent in writing was obtained from all participants or from close relatives. The local Medical Ethics Committee approved the study.

Design

Participants were randomly assigned to the experimental group or to the control group. The allocation sequence was computer generated and concealed in sequentially numbered opaque sealed envelopes until randomisation. The experimental group received 10–11 hours of treatment with Multicue in sessions of 30–45 minutes with a frequency of two to three times a week in a period of approximately 2 months. Apart from the assigned language therapy, no other therapy was allowed, except psychosocial group therapy aimed at coping with the consequences of aphasia. Treatment was delivered by the therapist who referred the participants. The control group received no treatment for 6–8 weeks.

Treatment

Multicue comprises four series of 80 pictures that are randomly presented. The program offers high and low frequency words of varying length (one to four syllables). A coloured picture is presented, and when the users are unable to find the target word, they may select one of the options in the main menu (see Figure 1 and Appendix B for more details):

- semantic cues: "Word meaning"
- orthographic cues: "Word form"
- sentence completion: "When do you use it"
- distraction: "Take a break"

While exploring these options, users are expected to check systematically what they already know about the meaning or form of the target word. As a second step, cues can be activated.

During the first four sessions, the therapist follows a protocol to familiarise the user with Multicue. In the first session, only the orthographic menu is activated. The other cues are introduced in the second and third sessions. In the fourth session, all cues are available and the user is encouraged to try as many cues as possible, in order to discover which cues are helpful. He or she is shown how to check whether the word is correct by selecting the button "I know the word". No specific response is required. Users may compare their spoken, written, or thought response with the computer-generated written target. When relevant, synonyms are supplied. When the user gives a correct written response, positive reinforcement is given.

After the fourth session, therapist involvement is reduced. However, he/she checks regularly how the participant progresses and whether the user is "stuck" on one particular cue that is not helpful (in which case this cue can be de-activated by the therapist).

To ensure correct application of the therapy programs, the researchers regularly discussed the content of therapy and problems of application with the therapists.

Assessment

Before and after therapy the participants were assessed by the researchers. The primary outcome measure was the Boston Naming Test (Kaplan, Goodglass, & Weintraub, 1983), consisting of 60 pictures. Some of our subjects had severe word finding problems and

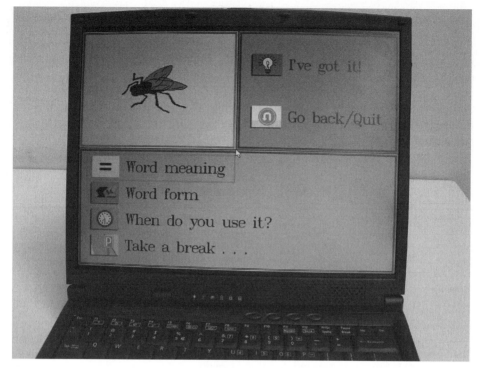

Figure 1. Multicue main menu.

were blocked during the administration of the test. In those cases, assessment could be terminated at 15 items, 30 items, or 45 items (pre- and post scores were based on the same number of items). Each response is scored on a 4-point rating scale (Van Loon-Vervoorn et al., 1995) (see Appendix A).

Verbal communicative ability was measured with the Amsterdam Nijmegen Everyday Language Test (ANELT, Blomert, Kean, Koster, & Schokker, 1994; Blomert, Koster, & Kean, 1995), scale A (Understandability). The ANELT-A is a valid and reliable measure in which verbal responses in 10 situations are scored on a 5-point scale for information content.

Statistics

We estimated that a sample size of 2×10 patients would provide a power of more than 70%, assuming a difference of 18 points in mean improvement on the BNT between the treated and the untreated group, and a standard deviation of 16.

The null hypothesis, i.e., no difference in mean improvement on the BNT and ANELT-A between the Multicue group and the no-treatment group, was tested with an independent samples t-test. T-based confidence intervals (CI) are reported.

Furthermore, the difference between pre- and post therapy scores on the BNT and ANELT-A was compared by means of a paired samples t-test for each group.

An alpha level of .05 was used for all statistical tests.

RESULTS

A total of 19 persons with aphasia entered the study; 10 were randomised to no treatment and 9 to Multicue. One participant in the Multicue group was lost to follow-up due to illness. The groups did not differ with respect to age, sex, handedness, time post onset, type and site of lesion, BNT-scores, ANELT-A scores, performance on the Weigl Sorting Test (a measure of executive functioning, Weigl, 1927), or content of previous treatment (semantic or phonological). See Table 1 for pretherapy characteristics of participants.

TABLE 1
Characteristics of participants

		Multicue (n = 8)	No treatment (n = 10)
Age	mean (sd)	62 (9)	65 (12)
Sex	Male	4	5
Time p.o. inclusion	mean (range)	13 (11–16) months	13 (11–17) months
Aetiology	infarction	7	10
	haemorrhage	1	
Site of stroke	left hemisphere	8	10
Handedness	right-handed	7	10
	left-handed	1	
BNT (max = 180)	mean (sd)	63 (37)	74 (35)
ANELT-A (max = 50)	mean (sd)	34 (9)	29 (12)
Previous treatment	semantic	5	5
	phonological	3	5
Executive function: Weigl Sorting Test (max = 15)	mean (sd)	6 (2)	5 (2)

BNT: Boston Naming Test. ANELT-A: Amsterdam-Nijmegen Everyday Language Test, scale A

TABLE 2
BNT and ANELT-A scores of participants who were randomised to Multicue (n = 8) and no treatment (n = 10)

	Multicue	No treatment		p
	mean (sd)	mean (sd)	t (df)	(2-tailed)
BNT score pre-treatment (max = 180)	63.1 (36.9)	74.0 (34.9)	0.64 (16)	0.53
BNT score post-treatment (max = 180)	75.6 (38.7)	75.7 (36.7)	0.00 (16)	1.0
BNT mean improvement	12.5 (11.8)	1.7 (17.4)	−1.50 (16)	0.15
ANELT-A score pre-treatment (max = 50)	33.9 (9.2)	28.6 (12.2)	−1.00 (16)	0.33
ANELT-A score post-treatment (max = 50)	34.3 (8.4)	25.5 (10.3)	−1.95 (16)	0.07
ANELT-A mean improvement	0.4 (4.0)	−3.1 (7.0)	−1.25 (16)	0.23

BNT: Boston Naming Test. ANELT-A: Amsterdam-Nijmegen Everyday Language Test, scale A

The mean BNT-score did not improve for the participants receiving no treatment, $t(9)$ = 0.31, p = .76 (2-tailed), but the participants receiving Multicue improved their scores significantly, $t(7)$ = 3.00, p = .02 (2-tailed). The mean ANELT-score did not improve for the participants who received no treatment, $t(9)$ = 1.40, p = .19 (2-tailed), nor for the participants receiving Multicue, $t(7)$ = 0.27, p = .80 (2-tailed). Mean improvement did not differ between the groups, neither for the BNT (95% CI: −4.5 to 26.1), nor for the ANELT-A (95% CI: −2.4 to 9.4) (see Table 2).

DISCUSSION

In this study, persons with chronic aphasia improved significantly on oral naming of untreated items (Boston Naming Test) after working with Multicue for a short period with minimal therapist involvement. Participants who received no treatment did not improve, and the comparison of the difference in improvement between treated and untreated participants suggested a beneficial effect of Multicue in this small study. The effect on oral naming was achieved by means of written cues and written feedback in therapy,[1] a cross-modal effect in line with previous findings (Deloche et al., 1992; Fink et al., 2002; Nickels, 2002; Van Mourik et al., 1992).

The question is, what is the underlying cause of the improvement, particularly whether the users had learned to cue themselves, or Multicue had improved the process of word finding. Our data do not provide an answer to this question, because the treatment protocol did not include detailed observations of participants during treatment and assessment. Moreover, self-cueing is difficult to assess, because it may occur without being observed in the speaker's behaviour. However, some single case studies report observations that support either interpretation of their findings.

A person with aphasia who learned to cue himself was described by Nickels (1992). He had better written naming than oral naming and was taught to find the first grapheme of a word and to pronounce the corresponding sound. Subsequently, the participant was encouraged to incorporate this grapheme–phoneme conversion skill into a naming strategy. The participant was observed to be overtly using the first phoneme as a self-cue after treatment.

On the other hand, Robson, Marshall, Pring, and Chiat (1998) reported a positive effect of a cueing treatment on the process of word finding. They encouraged their participant to reflect upon the syllabic structure and first phoneme of pictured targets. Subsequently, she was asked to use this partial phonological knowledge as a self-cue. Naming performance improved, also for untreated items. Because the participant was not observed to make use of self-cueing, neither overt nor covert (hesitations), the authors concluded that the treatment had led to improved phonological access, rather than an ability to self-cue.

Contrary to our hypothesis, improvement on the BNT did not generalise to verbal communication as measured with the ANELT-A. More sensitive measures may be needed to detect the effect of improved word finding on verbal communication, for instance the number of content words in conversation, a measure that was shown to be strongly related to picture naming (Hickin, Best, Herbert, Howard, & Osborne, 2001).

Alternatively, the gap between naming and verbal communication may be unbridgeable for some patients. It is increasingly recognised that non-linguistic cognitive deficits

---

[1] and perhaps written and/or oral naming: the user is not required to produce the word, but may choose to do so.

may have a large influence on the efficacy of aphasia therapy. Deficits in executive functioning are offered as possible explanations for why the abilities trained in therapy do not generalise to everyday life (Helm-Estabrooks & Ratner, 2000; Purdy, 2002). Non-linguistic cognitive deficits may certainly have played a role in our study; performance of the participants on a test of executive functioning (Weigl Sorting Test) was relatively low. These deficits may not only have prevented generalisation to everyday communication, but they may also have influenced the effect of Multicue on naming. The learning principle of Multicue, i.e., discovery-based learning, is likely to require more of users in terms of executive functioning than drill and practice. Users have to discover by themselves which cues are most useful to them. They have to keep the different cues and their effectiveness in memory and compare them, and flexibly shift to another cue when the chosen cue is not helpful. It is possible that many persons with aphasia who have poor executive functions would benefit more from an approach that requires less flexibility. Presenting the cues in a fixed order, and not asking the user to choose between different cues, but to check them all, may be a better approach for people with cognitive limitations. It may be easier to internalise a fixed procedure that can be used in communicative situations. This was observed by Christinaz (personal communication in Katz, 2001). Participants worked with a computer that displayed a fixed series of questions each time they experienced word finding problems. "Patients reported after several weeks of using the computer, that they no longer required it, instead asking themselves the same series of questions previously displayed by the computer. Christinaz reasoned that the participants had internalised the algorithm and now cued themselves without the need of external prompts." (Katz, 2001, p. 727). A study in which this approach (i.e., learning focused on internalising a fixed set of cues) is compared with the Multicue approach (i.e. discovery-based learning) may be relevant for clinical practice.

The results of our study are encouraging, especially in view of the fact that, although the participants were more than a year post stroke onset and had already received intensive impairment-oriented treatment, they further improved their naming ability with Multicue therapy. Moreover, this effect was found after only 10 hours of treatment. This is a minimal amount of therapy according to Bhogal, Teasell, and Speechley (2003), who in their review found that studies that showed an effect of aphasia therapy provided 93 (60–120) hours of therapy in 11 (8–12) weeks, whereas studies that showed no effect provided 44 hours (30–52) of therapy in 23 (20–26) weeks. Future studies need to establish whether more intensive Multicue treatment leads to larger effects on naming and possibly generalisation to verbal communication.

REFERENCES

Aftonomos, L. B., Appelbaum, J. S., & Steele, R. D. (1999). Improving outcomes for persons with aphasia in advanced community-based treatment programs. *Stroke, 30,* 1370–1379.

Avila, C., Lambon Ralph, M. A., Parcet, M-A., Geffner, D., & Gonzalez-Darder, J-M. (2001). Implicit word cues facilitate impaired naming performance: Evidence from a case of anomia. *Brain and Language, 79,* 185–200.

Basso, A., Marangolo, P., Piras, F., & Galluzzi, C. (2001). Acquisition of new "words" in normal subjects: A suggestion for the treatment of anomia. *Brain and Language, 77,* 45–59.

Bhogal, S. K., Teasell, R., & Speechley, M. (2003). Intensity of aphasia therapy, impact on recovery. *Stroke, 34,* 987–993.

Blomert, L., Kean, M. L., Koster, C., & Schokker, J. (1994). Amsterdam-Nijmegen Everyday Language Test: Construction, reliability and validity. *Aphasiology, 8,* 381–407.

Blomert, L., Koster, Ch., & Kean, M. L. (1995). *Amsterdam-Nijmegen Test voor Alledaagse Taalvaardigheid.* Lisse: Swets & Zeitlinger.

Boyle, M., & Coelho, C. A. (1995). Application of semantic feature analysis as a treatment for aphasic dysnomia. *American Journal of Speech-Language Pathology, 4*, 94–98.

Bruce, C., & Howard, D. (1987). Computer-generated phonemic cues: An effective aid for naming in aphasia. *British Journal of Disorders of Communication, 22*, 191–201.

Coelho, C. A., McHugh, R. E., & Boyle, M. (2000). Semantic feature analysis as a treatment for aphasic dysnomia: A replication. *Aphasiology, 14*, 133–142.

Colby, K., Christinaz, D., Parkinson, R., Graham, S., & Karpf, C. (1981). A word-finding computer program with a dynamic lexical-semantic memory for patients with anomia using an intelligent speech prosthesis. *Brain and Language, 14*, 272–281.

Deloche, G., Ferrand, I., Metz-Lutz, M-N., Dordain, M., Kremin, H., Hannequin, D., et al. (1992). Confrontation naming rehabilitation in aphasics: A computerised written technique. *Neuropsychological Rehabilitation, 2*, 117–124.

Doesborgh, S. J. C., van de Sandt-Koenderman, M. E., Dippel, D. W. J., van Harskamp, F., Koudstaal, P. J., & Visch-Brink, E. G. (2004). The effects of semantic treatment on verbal communication and linguistic processing in aphasia after stroke: A randomized controlled trial. *Stroke, 35*, 141–146.

Drew, R. L., & Thompson, C. K. (1999). Model-based semantic treatment for naming deficits in aphasia. *Journal of Speech, Language and Hearing Research, 42*, 972–989.

Fink, R. B., Brecher, A., Schwartz, M. F., & Robey, R. R. (2002). A computer-implemented protocol for treatment of naming disorders: Evaluation of clinician-guided and partially self-guided instruction. *Aphasiology, 16*, 1061–1086.

Franklin, S. E., Buerk, F., & Howard, D. (2002). Generalised improvement in speech production for a subject with reproduction conduction aphasia. *Aphasiology, 16*, 1087–1114.

Helm-Estabrooks, N., & Ratner, N. B. (2000). Executive functions: What are they, and why do they matter? Description, disorders, management. *Seminars in Speech and Language, 21*, 91–92.

Hickin, J., Best, W., Herbert, R., Howard, D., & Osborne, F. (2001). Treatment of word retrieval in aphasia: Generalisation to conversational speech. *International Journal of Language and Communication Disorders, 36*, 13–18.

Hickin, J., Best, W., Herbert, R., Howard, D., & Osborne, F. (2002a). Phonological therapy for word-finding difficulties: a re-evaluation. *Aphasiology, 16*, 981–999.

Hickin, J., Herbert, R., Best, W., Howard, D., & Osborne, F. (2002b). Efficacy of treatment: Effects on word retrieval and conversation. In S. Byng, C. Pound, & J. Marshall (Eds.), *The aphasia therapy file 2.* Hove, UK: Psychology Press.

Hillis, A. E. (1989). Efficacy and generalization of treatment for aphasic naming errors. *Archives of Physical Medicine and Rehabilitation, 70*, 632–636.

Howard, D., & Orchard-Lisle, V. (1984). On the origin of semantic errors in naming: Evidence from the case of a global aphasic. *Cognitive Neuropsychology, 1*, 163–190.

Kaplan, E., Goodglass, H., & Weintraub, S. (1983). *Boston Naming Test.* Philadelphia, PA: Lea & Febiger.

Katz, R-C. (2001). Computer applications in aphasia treatment. In R. Chapey (Ed.), *Language intervention strategies in aphasia and related neurogenic communication disorders* (4th ed.). Philadelphia: Lippincott Williams & Wilkins.

Kinsey, C. (1990). Analysis of dysphasics' behaviour in computer and conventional therapy environment. *Aphasiology, 4*, 281–291.

McNeil, M. R., Doyle, P. J., Spencer, K. A., Jackson Goda, A., Flores, D., & Small, S. L. (1997). A double-blind, placebo-controlled study of pharmacological and behavioural treatment of lexical-semantic deficits in aphasia. *Aphasiology, 11*, 385–400.

Nickels, L. A. (1992). The autocue? Self-generated phonemic cues in the treatment of a disorder of reading and naming. *Cognitive Neuropsychology, 9*, 155–182.

Nickels, L. A. (2002). Therapy for naming disorders: Revisiting, revising, and reviewing. *Aphasiology, 16*, 935–979.

Nickels, L., & Best, W. (1996). Therapy for naming disorders (Part II): Specifics, surprises and suggestions. *Aphasiology, 10*, 109–136.

Purdy, M. (2002). Executive function ability in persons with aphasia. *Aphasiology, 16*, 549–557.

Raymer, A. M., Thompson, C. K., Jacobs, B., & Le Grand, H. R. (1993). Phonological treatment of naming deficits in aphasia: Model-based generalization analysis. *Aphasiology, 7*, 27–53.

Robson, J., Marshall, J., Pring, T., & Chiat, S. (1998). Phonological naming therapy in jargon aphasia: Positive but paradoxical effects. *Journal of the International Neuropsychological Society, 4*, 675–686.

Stachowiak, F. J. (1993). Computer-based aphasia therapy with the Lingware/STACH system. In F. J. Stachowiak, R. De Bleser, G. Deloche, R. Kaschel, H. Kremin, P. North et al. (Eds.), *Developments in the assessment and rehabilitation of brain-damaged patients* (pp. 354–380). Tubingen: Gunter Narr Verlag.

Van de Sandt-Koenderman, W. M., & Visch-Brink, E. G. (1993). Experiences with Multicue. In F. J. Stachowiak, R. De Bleser, G. Deloche, R. Kaschel, H. Kremin, P. North et al. (Eds.), *Developments in the assessment and rehabilitation of brain-damaged patients* (pp. 347–351). Tubingen: Gunter Narr Verlag.

Van Loon-Vervoorn, W. A., Stumpel, H. J., & De Vries, L. A. (1995). Benoemingsproblemen bij links- en rechtzijdig hersenletsel. *Logopedie en Foniatrie, 2*, 35–41.

Van Mourik, M., & Van de Sandt-Koenderman, W. M. (1992). Multicue. *Aphasiology, 6*, 179–183.

Wambaugh, J., Linebaugh, C., Doyle, P., Martinez, A., Kalinyak-Fliszar, M., & Spencer, K. (2001). Effects of two cueing treatments on lexical retrieval in aphasic speakers with different levels of deficit. *Aphasiology, 15*, 933–950.

Weigl, E. (1927). Zur Psychologie sogenannter Abstraktionsprozesse. *Zeitschrift für Psychologie, 103*, 2–45.

APPENDIX A

Scoring Boston Naming Test

3 points = correct or correct with phonological or dysarthric distortion (at least 2/3 correct).

2 points = self-correction, long hesitation, correct word used in a sentence, semantically closely related word (e.g., category name / second part of a compound), good description.

1 point = semantically related word (unspecific category name / first part of a compound), reasonable description.

0 points = semantically unrelated word, bad description, neologism, automatism, perseveration, no response, avoidant phrase, wrong interpretation based on perceptual commonalities (including naming of a part of the picture).

APPENDIX B

Options and cues in Multicue

Main menu	Submenu
Word meaning	Features (e.g., form, category, function, location)
	Semantic associations
	Description
	Drawing (to be made by user)
Word form	First letter
	Number of syllables and stresspattern
	Last letter
Sentence completion ("When do you use it")	
Distraction ("Take a break")	(contains 11 melodies)

APHASIOLOGY, 2004, *18* (3), 223–228

Computers in aphasia therapy: Effects and side-effects

Claus-W. Wallesch

*Otto-von-Guericke University, and Institute of Neurological and
Neurosurgical Rehabilitation Research, Magdeburg, Germany*

Helga Johannsen-Horbach

School of Speech Therapy, Freiburg, Germany

We review published studies on the use of computers in aphasia therapy. Computer-based
treatment seems attractive, especially as it may allow for massed practice. We discuss
possible side-effects. Aphasia rehabilitation must aim at a reduction of handicap. At least
one published study described an improvement in functional communication after treatment with a comprehensive programme that included both therapist-delivered speech-
language therapy and home computer training. It cannot be decided to what extent functional communication-orientation of the programme, computer use, intensity of treatment,
or even other factors contributed to the positive effect, as no control group was included.
A randomised controlled trial with adequate control groups and adequate, handicap-
oriented outcome measurements is warranted to evaluate the effectiveness of the computer
component and its effect size.

Computer-based therapeutic approaches have been demonstrated as beneficial in the
treatment of attention and memory disorders (e.g., Grealy, Johnson, & Rushton, 1999),
visual field defects (e.g., Kasten, Wust, Behrens-Baumann, & Sabel, 1998), and hemi-
neglect (e.g., Webster, McFarland, Rapport, Morrill, Roades, & Abadee, 2001). For these
deficits of patient-centred instrumental functions, the correlation between disability and
handicap is close. However, even treatment of these impairments can be improved by use
of "virtual reality" (Ring, 1998). In the case of aphasia therapy, virtual reality would
constitute an interactive communicative environment. Although massive technological
advances are occurring at a rapid pace, a breakthrough has yet to occur for man–computer
communication.

In most instances, computer-assisted treatments are either tailored or responsive to the
patient's individual requirements, and most of them include strategies of massed practice/
forced use (Taub, Miller, Novack, Cook, Fleming, Nepomuceno, et al., 1993). The
computer is being used a therapeutic tool employed by a (competent) therapist for the
attainment of individual and specified goals (a notable exception is Katz & Wertz, 1997,
who minimised therapists' activities).

Address correspondence to: Prof. Dr Claus-W.Wallesch, Department of Neurology, Otto-von-Guericke-
University, Leipziger Str. 44, 39120 Magdeburg, Germany. Email: neuro.wallesch@medizin.uni-magdeburg.de

Work on this review was supported by the Research Program on Rehabilitation Sciences Sachsen-Anhalt/
Mecklenburg-Vorpommern of the Federal Ministry of Education and Research and the German Statutory
Pension Funds (CW) and the Deutsche Angestellten Akademie (HJH).

http://www.tandf.co.uk/journals/pp/02687038.html   DOI: 10.1080/02687030444000039

MASSED PRACTICE/ FORCED USE

Massed practice and forced use have been demonstrated to result in rearrangements of cortical representations (Liepert, Uhde, Gräf, Leidner, & Weiller, 2001). Obviously, computers are an appropriate instrument to apply massed practice. They possess technological appeal, are discreet, and never bored. However, the question arises of what constitutes massed practice for an aphasic person. We are convinced that drill alone does not suffice.

It has been demonstrated in a randomised study that massed practice together with forced verbal communication results in improvements of communication performance of chronic aphasics in comparison to standard neurolinguistically oriented speech therapy with lower intensity but the same absolute amount of treatment hours (Pulvermüller, Neininger, Elbert, Mohr, Rockstroh, Koebbel, et al., 2001). This is not trivial, as most effects of aphasia therapy have been documented as improvements in test performance only. However, it cannot be unequivocally determined whether the convincing effect on communicative behaviour was due to the intensity or the type of treatment, i.e., its focus on verbal communicative acts. The latter focus may have biased measurements on the Communication Activity Log and on blinded ratings of communication behaviour, both of which were used as outcome measures. Pulvermüller et al. propose three principles of aphasia therapy, namely massed practice, constraint induction, and behavioural relevance. Their study demonstrates that at least one of these is relevant. However, it does not unequivocally indicate which.

VARIABLES INFLUENCING TREATMENT EFFECTIVENESS

It has been demonstrated that the effectiveness of (more conventional) treatment is influenced by numerous individual (linguistic and nonlinguistic) variables (e.g., Hillis, 1998). Computer-based neurolinguistic therapy should therefore be able to address these variables on an individualised basis, which again would require its application by a competent diagnostician/ therapist.

A direct correlation between measured gains in treatment and social validity has not yet been demonstrated (compare Jacobs, 2001). This problem, of course, affects both computer-based and conventional therapy. For patient and family, it is important to engage their limited (attentional, motivational) resources in a way that promises greatest improvements in their quality of life, which is dominated by social functions. Communicative impairment is not the most disabling of the patients' handicaps as judged by patients and their close others (Herrmann & Wallesch, 1989; Wenz & Herrmann, 1990).

ADVANTAGES AND SIDE-EFFECTS OF COMPUTER-BASED THERAPY

According to Katz and Wertz (1997, p. 494):

> Computers can be powerful clinical tools. They can be used to administer activities designed by clinicians and to measure patient performance. Sophisticated programs can modify stimulus and response characteristics, provide cues, and change tasks in response to patient performance. Computers have the potential for increasing the amount of time patients are involved in treatment and providing more treatment at lower cost.

In 1992, Matthews, Harley, and Malec described risks and side-effects of the use of computers in neuropsychological treatment. Among others, their guidelines address the following issues:

(1) Does computer-assisted cognitive rehabilitation have a role in the practice of clinical neuropsychology?

"Appropriate clinical use of computer software in rehabilitation is dependent upon maintaining a clear distinction between software being properly viewed as a component in an organized treatment program versus being improperly viewed as treatment itself" (p. 122).

We conclude that the treatment strategy must generate training (sub)goals, the attainment of which can be facilitated by the use of an appropriate computer program.

(2) Consumer protection, risk/benefit analysis:

"One potential risk of cognitive rehabilitation is that false hopes may be raised, and denial of disability may be reinforced (...). A second risk is that the development of an isolated or task-specific skill may serve as false evidence of general competency (...). This can interfere with rehabilitation efforts and recommendations for safe conduct. Generalization must be demonstrated and not merely presumed. Thirdly, focusing efforts and time in the use of cognitive rehabilitation software runs the risk of diverting attention from more problematic concerns which potentially may be more directly remediable. These would include family problems, social and vocational adjustment issues, emotional disorders, and financial problems. (...) Fourth, significant time spent working with cognitive rehabilitation software may perpetuate social isolation (...). Risks can be reduced by the use of computer-assisted and other cognitive rehabilitation procedures in the context of an organized treatment program" (Matthews et al., 1992, p. 126).

The necessity of a treatment strategy aiming at a reduction of handicap is reinforced. Matthews et al. voice their concern that even an improvement in (test) performance may coincide with detrimental social effects and thus an increase in overall handicap. Their focus on social effects is important. Research on caregiver burden demonstrates that social isolation negatively affects their quality of life (Scholte op Reimer, de Haan, Rijnders, Limburg, & van den Bos, 1998). The problem of possible negative social effects of computer therapy in aphasia has been addressed by Petheram (1996) who found no evidence of harmful behaviour.

COMPUTER USE IN APHASIA REHABILITATION

Computerised aids

Computers can be employed in different ways for aphasia rehabilitation. They may be used as an aid to improve communication, similar to their employment as an externalised memory store for people with amnesia (Wright, Rogers, Hall, Wilson, Evans, Emslie, et al., 2001). The C-VIC (Computerized Visual Communication) system is an iconic communication device that uses the unique features available with the use of computers, such as animated symbols (Weinrich, 1997). "Most remarkable, however, is the generalization of C-VIC trainings to improvements in English production. Some patients with chronic, severe expressive aphasia demonstrate significant improvements in their English production of active sentences" (Weinrich, McCall, Weber, Thomas, & Thornburg, 1995, p. 362). Without the use of computers, a similar generalisation effect has been reported by Johannsen-Horbach, Cegla, Mager, Schempp, and Wallesch (1985) when employing a symbol language in the treatment of chronic severe nonfluent aphasics. Iconic communication systems are used as a communication approach for patients with aphasia and their partners only under very rare circumstances. Computer devices with spoken language output (or even input) may, however, greatly facilitate symbol-based communication. We still doubt that significant numbers of patients with aphasia will have both the deficit pattern and the skills together with the necessary acceptance and compliance to use such tools. The use of a computer device to prompt and substitute word finding and sentence generation in severely nonfluent aphasics has been investigated by Waller, Dennis, Brodie, and Cairns (1998) with mixed results.

Improvement of specific functions and the question of generalisation

Of special interest to the topic is the study of Katz and Wertz (1997), as they were able to demonstrate generalisation effects. Only reading skills were trained 3 hours per week for 26 weeks. The study included a control group which was stimulated by nonverbal computer games and cognitive rehabilitation tasks. The investigation addressed the following questions:

- Can computerised reading treatment be administered with minimal assistance from a clinician? (Answer: Yes, when the program adapts to patient performance.)
- Is computer reading treatment for chronic aphasic patients efficacious? (Answer: Questionable, generalisation effects were demonstrated only in tests PICA and WAB.)
- Does improvement on computer reading tasks generalise to non-computer reading performance? (Answer: Yes.)
- Does improvement result from the language content of the software and not simply by stimulation provided by a computer? (Answer: Yes, as shown by comparison with control group.)

The computer reading group exhibited significant improvement on the Porch Index of Communicative Ability "Overall" and "Verbal" modalities and on the Western Aphasia Battery "Aphasia Quotient" and "Repetition" performance. The authors thus were able to demonstrate that computerised reading treatment generalises to non-computer non-written language use. It remains unresolved whether communicative performance was improved.

Might the use of computerised tasks within a therapeutic strategy improve communication?

Aftonomos, Applebaum, and Steele (1999) investigated patients with aphasia enrolled in two community-based therapy programmes, which use a specifically designed computer-based tool that is employed therapeutically in adherence to an extensive, detailed, and formally trained patient care algorithm. Participants received an average of 2 hours of (therapist-delivered) treatment per week for 4–47 weeks. They were not selected for aphasia syndrome and on the average were 2 years post onset (more than 75% > 6 months). There was no control group.

According to Aftonomos et al. (1999, p. 1372):

> During treatment, focus was invariably on improving patients' functional communication outside the clinic, as opposed to training for higher scores on discharge testing. When patient responses in therapy sessions so indicate, batteries of exercises are loaded onto the patient's system as prescribed home practice. At home, patients are to complete the prescribed clinical exercises, and additionally they may pursue materials of their own choosing, explore

semantic domains to review lexical items within, or find other activities that engage their interest. Analysis has shown that patients typically engage in such self-directed activities approximately 2 hours per day.

Thus, the programme does not include forced use, but certainly massed practice.

The authors were able to show a significant improvement of both acute (< 6 months post onset) and chronic (> 6 months post onset) on the Communicative Effectiveness Index (Lomas, Pickard, Bester, Elbard, Finlayson, & Zoghaib, 1989). However, it cannot be extracted from the data whether the improvement was due to the availability, quality, or intensity of treatment, or specifically to the use of the computer software.

SUMMARY AND CONCLUSION

The question of "ecological validity", i.e., the reduction of handicap, has not yet been answered for any type of aphasia therapy. An abundance of single case and uncontrolled small group studies suggest that aphasia therapy is effective with respect to an improvement of language functions, and a meta-analysis that did not use the rigorous selection criteria of the Cochrane Collaboration evaluated aphasia therapy positively (Robey, 1994). As it is very difficult to assess language-related impairment of quality of life, measured, assessed, or observed changes of communicative behaviour must suffice as the gold-standard of therapeutic success for the time being.

Both the Aftonomos et al. (1999) and the Pulvermüller et al. (2001) studies included assessments of communicative functions, and both demonstrated improvements after treatment. However, neither study shows which element of therapy contributed to the effect. Intensity of treatment could be the decisive factor for both treatment approaches or, alternatively, their focus on communication performance. Outside highly artificial "micro worlds" actual communication with a computer system is still not possible, therefore a focus on communication is difficult to realise with artificial intelligence.

Computer-based therapy can have important advantages for the application of massed practice. Programs can be designed to respond to patient performance (e.g., adapt difficulty, change after criterion is reached, etc.), the graphics and media support are overwhelming, and so on. In our experience, many patients and spouses want "massed practice" and spend many hours with "homework", regardless of whether this has been assigned by the therapist or not. We doubt the therapeutic sense of most of these types of homework, and see in patient and partner doing homework together a further strain and potential burden on their relationship. Here, computerised therapy could provide a better integration into the therapeutic strategy and control of these home activities by the therapist, and could ease strain and implicit demands on partners.

We were impressed by the stringent therapeutic structure of the approach described by Aftonomos et al. (1999) that integrates computer homework and volunteer activities into a strategic algorithm. However, a randomised controlled trial with adequate control groups and adequate outcome measurements is warranted to evaluate the effectiveness of the computer component and its effect size.

REFERENCES

Aftonomos, L. B., Appelbaum, J. S., & Steele, R. D. (1999). Improving outcomes for persons with aphasia in advanced community-based treatment programs. *Stroke, 30*, 1370–1379.

Grealy, M. A., Johnson, D. A., & Rushton, S. K. (1999). Improving cognitive function after brain injury: The use of exercise and virtual reality. *Archives of Physical Medicine and Rehabilitation, 80*, 661–667.

Herrmann, M., & Wallesch, C. W. (1989). Psychosocial changes and psychosocial adjustment with chronic and severe nonfluent aphasia. *Aphasiology, 3*, 513–526.

Hillis, A. E. (1998). Treatment of naming disorders: New issues regarding old therapies. *Journal of the International Neuropsychological Society, 4*, 648–660.

Jacobs, B. J. (2001). Social validity of changes in informativeness and efficiency of aphasic discourse following linguistic specific treatment (LST). *Brain and Language, 78*, 115–127.

Johannsen-Horbach, H., Cegla, B., Mager, U., Schempp, B., & Wallesch, C. W. (1985). Treatment of chronic global aphasia with a nonverbal communication system. *Brain and Language, 24*, 74–82.

Kasten, E., Wust, S., Behrens-Baumann, W., & Sabel, B. A. (1998). Computer-based training for the treatment of partial blindness. *Nature Medicine, 4*, 1005–1006.

Katz, R. C., & Wertz, R. T. (1997). The efficacy of computer-provided reading treatment for chronic aphasic adults. *Journal of Speech, Language and Hearing Research, 40*, 493–507.

Liepert, J., Uhde, I., Gräf, S., Leidner, O., & Weiller, C. (2001). Motor cortex plasticity during forced-use therapy in stroke patients: A preliminary study. *Journal of Neurology, 248*, 315–321.

Lomas, J., Pickard, L., Bester, S., Elbard, H., Finlayson, A., & Zoghaib, C. (1989). The Communicative Effectiveness Index: Development and psychometric evaluation of a functional measure of adult aphasia. *Journal of Speech and Hearing Disorders, 154*, 113–124.

Matthews, C. G., Harley, J. P., & Malec, J. F. (1992). Guidelines for computer-assisted neuropsychological rehabilitation and cognitive remediation. In K. M. Adams & B. P. Rourke (Eds.), *The TCN guide to professional practice in clinical neuropsychological* (pp. 120–136). Amsterdam: Swets & Zeitlinger.

Petheram, B. (1996). The behaviour of stroke patients in unsupervised computer-administered aphasia therapy. *Disability & Rehabilitation, 18*, 21–26.

Pulvermüller, F., Neininger, B., Elbert, T., Mohr, B., Rockstroh, B., Koebbel, P., et al. (2001). Constraint-induced therapy of chronic aphasia. *Stroke, 32*, 1621–1626.

Ring, H. (1998). Is neurological rehabilitation ready for "immersion" in the world of virtual reality? *Disability & Rehabilitation, 20*, 98–101.

Robey, R. R. (1994). The efficacy of treatment for aphasic persons: A meta-analysis. *Brain and Language, 47*, 582–608.

Scholte op Reimer, W. J. M., de Haan, R. J., Rijnders, P. T., Limburg, M., & van den Bos, G. A. M. (1998). The burden of caregiving in partners of long-term stroke survivors. *Stroke, 29*, 1605–1611.

Taub, E., Miller, N. E., Novack, T. A., Cook, E. W., Fleming, W. D., Nepomuceno, C. S., et al. (1993). Technique to improve chronic motor deficit after stroke. *Archives of Physical Medicine and Rehabilitation, 74*, 347–354.

Waller, A., Dennis, F., Brodie, J., & Cairns, A. Y. (1998). Evaluating the use of TalksBac, a predictive communication device for nonfluent adults with aphasia. *International Journal of Language and Communication Disorders, 33*, 45–70.

Webster, J. S., McFarland, P. T., Rapport, L. J., Morrill, B., Roades, L. A., & Abadee, P. S. (2001). Computer-assisted training for improving wheelchair mobility in unilateral neglect patients. *Archives of Physical Medicine and Rehabilitation, 82*, 769–775.

Weinrich, M. (1997). Computer rehabilitation in aphasia. *Clinical Neuroscience, 4*, 103–107.

Weinrich, M., McCall, D., Weber, C., Thomas, K., & Thornburg, L. (1995). Training on an iconic communication system for severe aphasia can improve natural language production. *Aphasiology, 9*, 343–365.

Wenz, C., & Herrmann, M. (1990). Emotionales Erleben und subjektive Krankheitswahrnehmung bei chronischer Aphasie – ein Vergleich zwischen Patienten und deren Familienangehörigen. *Psychotherapie, Psychosomatik und Medizinische Psychologie, 40*, 488–495.

Wright, P., Rogers, N., Hall, C., Wilson, B., Evans, J., Emslie, H., et al. (2001). Comparison of pocket computer memory aids for people with brain injury. *Brain Injury, 15*, 787–800.

APHASIOLOGY, 2004, *18* (3), 229–244

Outcomes of computer-provided treatment for aphasia

Robert T. Wertz

VA Medical Center and Vanderbilt University School of Medicine, Nashville, TN, USA

Richard C. Katz

VA Medical Center, Phoenix, and Arizona State University, Tempe, AZ, USA

Background: Computers have become a familiar component of aphasia treatment over the past 20 years. Published research continues to indicate the influence computerised treatment may have on improving language performance of aphasic adults. As a result of the move to develop evidenced-based clinical guidelines, there is a need to evaluate the research methodology and the level of evidence provided by computerised interventions for aphasia.

Aims: The purposes of this paper are to evaluate examples of reports in the computerised treatment for aphasia outcomes research literature by applying precise definitions of the treatment outcome research terminology, placing the examples within the context of the five-phase treatment outcomes research model, applying a level of evidence scale to rate the evidence provided by the selected examples, and speculating where we are and where we may need to go in demonstrating the influence of computer-provided treatment on improvement in aphasia.

Methods & Procedures: We applied Robey and Schultz's (1998) model for conducting clinical-outcome research in aphasia and the level of evidence scale developed by the American Academy of Neurology (1994) to the results of computer-provided aphasia treatment studies. Eight Phase 1 studies, three series of Phase 2 studies, and one Phase 3 study are described as examples.

Outcomes & Results: While several Phase 1 and 2 studies imply that computer-provided treatment is active in the treatment of people with aphasia, evidence to support the efficacy of computerised treatment for adults with aphasia is based on a single Phase 3 study. Additional Phase 3 studies are needed to demonstrate the efficacy of additional treatment software, and Phase 4 and Phase 5 studies are necessary to demonstrate the effectiveness and efficiency of computerised treatment for people with aphasia.

The influence of computer-provided treatment on improvement in aphasia remains controversial. Robinson (1990) observed that the efficacy of computerised treatment for aphasia, as well as for other cognitive disorders, had not been demonstrated. Conversely, Katz and Wertz (1997) concluded that the computer-provided reading treatment they employed with their chronic aphasic participants was efficacious. Differences of opinion have resulted, perhaps, from failure to define the treatment outcomes research terminology—outcome, efficacy, effectiveness, efficiency; specify the appropriate research designs to demonstrate the influence of computer-provided treatment on outcome; and employ a level of evidence scale to evaluate reports of computerised treatment studies for aphasia.

Address correspondence to: Robert T. Wertz PhD, Audiology and Speech Pathology (126), VA Medical Center, 1310 24th Avenue South, Nashville, TN 37212, USA. Email: robert.wertz@med.va.gov

http://www.tandf.co.uk/journals/pp/02687038.html   DOI: 10.1080/02687030444000048

Robey and Schultz (1998) have provided a model for conducting clinical-outcome research that includes precise definitions of the outcomes research terminology and the application of the five-phase model for conducting treatment outcome research. Moreover, a level of evidence scale (American Academy of Neurology, 1994) is available to rate the results of computer-provided aphasia treatment studies. The purposes of this paper are to evaluate examples of reports in the computerised treatment for aphasia outcomes research literature by applying precise definitions of the treatment outcomes research terminology, placing the examples within the context of the five-phase treatment outcomes research model, applying a level of evidence scale to rate the evidence provided by the selected examples, and speculating where we are and where we may need to go in demonstrating the influence of computer-provided treatment on improvement in aphasia.

EVALUATING TREATMENT OUTCOME RESEARCH

As indicated above, precise definitions and uniform methods have not been applied in evaluation of computer-provided aphasia treatment outcome research. In addition, there has been no attempt to determine the level of evidence provided by specific reports on computer interventions. Thus, the absence of some "rules to live by" in conducting computer-provided treatment has hampered evaluation of the empirical evidence. Applying Robey and Schultz's (1998) definitions of the treatment outcomes terminology, their elaboration of the five-phase treatment outcome research model, and the American Academy of Neurology's (1994) level of evidence scale may bring some order to what has been a confusing endeavour.

Outcome research terminology

Failure to define the treatment outcome research terminology has led to a general, but inferentially naïve, impression that all treatment intervention investigations are a test of a treatment's efficacy. The terms "outcome", "efficacy", "effectiveness", and "efficiency" have been used inappropriately as synonyms. They are not, and assuming that they are creates confusion. While all terms fall under a general heading of "outcomes" research, specific conditions must be met to demonstrate "efficacy", "effectiveness", and "efficiency". In this report, we will apply the following definitions.

Outcome.   Robey and Schultz (1998, p. 789) observe:

> The terms clinical outcome research, treatment outcome research, or simply outcome research are variously invoked in the general community of clinical researchers to describe research designed to index (using valid and reliable measures) differences between experimental observations made prior to the implementation of a certain treatment protocol and observations made some time after the conclusion of that treatment (Sederer et al., 1996). Experimentation designed to assess the efficacy of a particular treatment is but one form of clinical-outcome research.

Thus, a treatment outcome is determined by comparing performance between two points in time, pre-treatment and post-treatment. Unless specific conditions are met, a treatment outcome indicates nothing about the efficacy, effectiveness, or efficiency of the treatment provided.

A straightforward, computer-provided treatment outcome study might select a sample of people with aphasia, document their performance pre-treatment with a specified outcome measure, administer a computerised treatment, re-evaluate performance post-treatment with the outcome measure, and compare the group's pre- and post-treatment performance. This process provides a simple outcome—group performance improved, got worse, or remained the same following the provision of treatment. The single group design will permit no inference about the treatment's efficacy, effectiveness, or efficiency. Inference is limited to speculation about the treatment's activity. If group performance improved significantly from pre- to post-treatment, the treatment may be active. If group performance remained the same or got worse, the treatment would be considered inactive.

Efficacy.   Robey and Schultz (1998) provide the Office of Technology Assessment's (OTA) (1978) definition of efficacy. The OTA defines efficacy as, "The probability of benefit to individuals in a defined population from a medical technology applied for a given medical problem under ideal conditions of use" (p. 16). The constraints inherent in the OTA definition are: inference about efficacy is applicable to a population, not an individual; the treatment and population are clearly specified; and the conditions under which efficacy is determined are optimal. Thus, as Robey and Schultz caution, because efficacy is demonstrated under ideal conditions, efficacy indicates the possible benefits of a treatment, not the actual benefits of a treatment.

The typical efficacy experiment is a randomised clinical trial in which study patients who meet selection criteria are assigned randomly to treatment and no-treatment groups. Pre-treatment performance is measured in both groups; the treatment group receives the treatment, and the no-treatment group is followed without treatment; and at the end of the treatment trial, both groups are re-evaluated. If the treatment group makes significantly more improvement than the no-treatment group, one can infer that the treatment was efficacious. Other requirements in an efficacy study are delivery of the treatment under ideal conditions—ideal treatment candidates, ideally trained therapists, ideal dosage (intensity and duration of treatment), and ideal outcome measures. Again, because of the ideal conditions, an efficacy experiment indicates whether a treatment can work, not whether it does work in actual conditions of clinical practice.

Effectiveness.   As with efficacy, Robey and Schultz (1998) provide the OTA (1978) definition of effectiveness. It is, "The probability of benefit to individuals in a defined population applied for a given medical problem under average conditions of use" (p. 16). Thus, while treatment efficacy research is designed to determine whether a treatment can work, treatment effectiveness research is designed to determine whether a treatment does work under everyday conditions. In efficacy studies, the conditions, as indicated above, are ideal. In effectiveness studies, the conditions are typical—typical patients, typical clinicians, typical intensity and duration of treatment, typical patient compliance, etc.

A rule of effectiveness research is that it is conducted only after a treatment has been demonstrated to be efficacious. Thus, a typical effectiveness study would employ a large, single group design that would test the effectiveness of a previously demonstrated efficacious treatment under conditions of daily practice. Performance would be evaluated pre-treatment, the treatment would be administered under ordinary conditions, and performance would be evaluated post-treatment. If significant improvement occurred from pre- to post-treatment, the treatment would be considered to be effective.

Efficiency.   Another term that is used in treatment outcomes research is efficiency. Wertz and Irwin (2001) define efficiency as, "acting or producing effectively with a minimum of waste, expense, or unnecessary effort, essentially, exhibiting a high ratio of output to input'' (p. 236). Efficiency studies can be a comparison of treatment designs to determine which of two treatments that have been demonstrated to be efficacious is the most efficient—i.e., achieves the most improvement with the same intensity and duration, or achieves similar improvement with less intensity and duration. Similarly, an efficiency study might compare the same treatment delivered on different schedules to determine whether the same outcome could be achieved with less duration and/or less intensity.

Five-phase treatment outcome research model

Robey and Schultz (1998) suggest that treatment outcome research should be program-matic—evolving systematically through each phase in the traditional five-phase outcome research model. They specify the purposes of each phase, how the treatment outcome terms apply in different phases, and the appropriate research designs for accomplishing the purposes in each phase. We consider each phase, briefly, below.

Phase 1. Purposes in Phase 1 are to develop the hypothesis about the treatment that will be tested in later phases in the model; establish the treatment's safety; and detect whether the treatment is active—essentially, whether people with aphasia who receive it improve. The studies are brief, employ small samples, and do not require external con-trols. Thus, small, single group and single subject designs are appropriate.

An example of a Phase 1 study might be examining the hypothesis that a computer-presented, hierarchical, word-retrieval programme will improve anomia in people with aphasia. A small sample of people with aphasia is selected, and their performance on word retrieval outcome measures is documented pre-treatment. The computer-presented, hierarchical, word-retrieval programme is administered, and after each participant completes the programme, post-treatment performance on the pre-treatment word-retrieval outcome measures is obtained. Comparison is made between the pre- and post-treatment performance. If post-treatment performance is significantly better than pre-treatment performance, the investigator may infer that the treatment may be active, and continue to Phase 2 studies. Safety issues would involve determining whether the treatment does more good than harm. In the behavioural, computerised treatment described above, the examiners would examine the number of adverse effects in the study sample and consider whether performance on the outcome measures deteriorated from pre- to post-treatment for any participants.

Phase 2. Purposes in Phase 2 are to refine the hypothesis developed in Phase 1, develop an explanation for why the treatment may be beneficial, specify the target population, standardise the treatment protocol, demonstrate the validity and reliability of the outcome measures, and determine the optimal dosage. As in Phase 1, Phase 2 studies are brief, employ small samples, and do not require external controls. Thus, small, single group and single subject designs are appropriate.

To satisfy the purposes of Phase 2 research, a series of studies may be necessary. For example, in the computer intervention described above in Phase 1, the investigator may refine his or her hypothesis by considering the stimuli. Are the stimuli more appropriate when auditory and visual modalities are combined than when either alone, auditory or visual, is employed? And is the hierarchy appropriately ordered; essentially, do the steps in the hierarchy lead progressively to the participants attaining the target behaviour? Are steps missing in the hierarchy? Phase 2 studies would employ a series of comparisons of the stimulus conditions—auditory, visual, and auditory-visual. Similarly, sequential performance by study participants would be examined to determine whether the hierarchy is appropriately ordered. Inordinate failure in moving from one step to another may suggest that steps are missing. Thus, a Phase 2 study might require an expanded hierarchy with a small group of participants.

To develop an explanation of why the treatment may be beneficial, the investigator could peruse the models of aphasia treatment provided by Horner, Loverso, and Gonzalez Rothi (1994). Comparison of the computer-provided treatment with the models may indicate a best fit is with the stimulation-facilitation model espoused by Schuell, Jenkins, and Jimenz Pabon (1964) and elaborated by Duffy and Coelho (2001). Thus, the premise for why the treatment may be beneficial is that language is an integrative activity that is linked to sensory and motor modalities but cannot be considered bound to them. In addition, intensive auditory and visual stimulation, provided by the computerised treatment, that includes meaningful material, abundant and varied stimuli, repetitive sensory stimulation, a response for each stimulus, under conditions where responses are elicited and not forced, provides the rationale for why the treatment may be beneficial.

Specifying the target population requires Phase 2 studies that identify the "ideal" study participants who will be selected in Phase 3, efficacy research. The investigator has an idea of the general target population from Phase 1 research. In Phase 2, a list of selection criteria is verified to identify study participants who are most likely to benefit from the treatment. These might include specification of age, education, aetiology, hearing and vision acuity, time post-onset, acceptable comorbidity, etc. After the list is compiled, it requires testing in Phase 2 small group or single subject research experiments to ensure that the selection criteria do, indeed, identify "ideal" participants—those who improve the most in the Phase 2 experiments.

Demonstrating the validity and reliability of the outcome measures requires that they measure what they report to measure—validity—and that they have acceptable intra- and inter-judge reliability. One seeks to measure change in the study participants and not change in the investigators. Moreover, in treatment outcome research, one wants to ensure the measures are sensitive in detecting change in performance from pre- to post-treatment if change occurs. And the investigator needs to consider whether the outcome measures will be acceptable to the scientific community for whom the results are intended.

Finally, Phase 2 research is necessary to determine the optimal dosage; intensity and duration of the treatment. This requires small group or single subject experiments that block on both, for example, length and number of sessions per week and number of weeks. One should eschew the heuristic assumption that "more is better" and let the empirical evidence indicate how much over what duration is best.

Phase 3.   The results of Phase 1 and 2 research must justify a test of the treatment's efficacy in Phase 3 under optimal conditions. The investigator has the data from Phase 1 and 2 studies to support what is "ideal"—study participants, clinician training, outcome measures, and dosage. Phase 3, efficacy studies are expensive. Large sample size is required to obtain acceptable statistical power, and, usually, the means for obtaining the large sample size is a multi-centre effort in which several institutions contribute participants in a collaborative effort. The required study design is a randomised clinical trial in which participants who meet selection criteria are assigned randomly to a treatment or no-treatment group. Randomisation controls for treatment selection bias and other potential biases, and the treatment versus no-treatment comparison constitutes a true test of the treatment's efficacy. Of course, tight control across participating centres is essential to ensure that the trial is truly cooperative—that everyone is doing the same thing.

Phase 4. If the treatment is demonstrated to be efficacious in Phase 3 efficacy research, it is justifiable to continue with Phase 4 effectiveness research. The purpose is to test the treatment's effectiveness under ordinary conditions of clinical practice with typical patients, typically trained clinicians, typical dosage, and typical compliance. Again, a large sample is required; however external control (e.g., a no-treatment control group) is not. Thus, the typical effectiveness study design is a large single group in which, as in Phase 1 research, performance is measured pre-treatment, the treatment is administered under ordinary conditions, performance is measured post-treatment, and a pre- versus post-treatment comparison is made to determine improvement. If the group shows significant improvement from pre- to post-treatment, one can infer that the treatment is effective—essentially, that it does work under conditions of everyday clinical practice.

Additional Phase 4 experiments might include examination of variations in the target population, for example, study participants who do not meet the selection criteria employed in the Phase 3 efficacy study. In addition, Phase 4 research might examine variation in the dosage, for example, a different intensity and duration of treatment from that employed in the Phase 3 efficacy research. And one might explore differences in treatment providers; for example, clinicians with less training than those who participated in the Phase 3 efficacy research or, perhaps, provision of the treatment by non-professional, trained volunteers.

Phase 5. Effectiveness research is continued in Phase 5, and studies may be initiated to test the treatment's efficiency. Continued effectiveness research might examine the cost-benefit, or cost-effectiveness, of the treatment. Or additional outcome measures might be employed to determine the patient's and family's satisfaction with the intervention or the influence of the treatment on the patient's quality of life. Large group studies and/or single subject designs with multiple replications across patients are appropriate for Phase 5 research and, usually, external control is not required. However, some efficiency studies require control through random assignment. For example, comparing the efficiency of two treatments that have been demonstrated to be efficacious in Phase 3 research requires a comparison of treatments design, where study participants who meet selection criteria are assigned randomly to one treatment or the other. Similarly, an efficiency study designed to compare one intensity and/or duration with another intensity and/or duration would require random assignment of study participants to the different schedules.

Level of evidence scale

A means for evaluating the results of treatment outcome research is the use of a level of evidence scale. Typically, these scales designate the quality of evidence available with a numerical—I, II, III—or alphabetical—A, B, C—system. Each level specifies the source of the evidence—randomised controlled trial, case control, cohort study, expert opinion, historical control, or case report.

A level of evidence scale, appropriate for evaluating computer-provided aphasia treatment research, has been developed by the American Academy of Neurology (1994). It specifies the following three levels of evidence.

Class I: Evidence from one or more well-designed, randomised, controlled clinical trials.

Class II: Evidence from one or more randomised clinical studies such as case-control, cohort studies, etc.

Class III: Evidence from expert opinion, non-randomised historical controls, or one or more case reports.

The scale is used to rate individual outcome research reports to determine the level of evidence provided. For example, a Phase 3 efficacy study that assigned study participants randomly to treatment and no-treatment groups, and observed that the treated group made significantly more improvement than the no-treatment group, would constitute Class I evidence. A non-randomised study that compared improvement in treated patients with improvement made by self-selected patients who did not receive treatment, and observed that the group who received treatment made significantly more improvement than the self-selected group that did not receive treatment, would demonstrate Class III evidence. Thus, application of the scale to the body of treatment literature would provide an evaluation of independent treatment studies and, collectively, give an impression of the value of the total evidence in demonstrating whether treatment, in general, may have an influence on improvement in aphasia.

We suggest caution in applying the "gold-standard" of a "randomised, controlled trial", because not all randomised controlled trials are created equal. For example, a randomised controlled trial that assigns study participants randomly to treatment and no-treatment groups is a direct test of a treatment's efficacy, and if positive results are obtained—treated participants make significantly more improvement than participants who receive no treatment—the study would provide Class I evidence. However, a randomised trial that compares two treatments of unknown efficacy lacks control for time and other variables and would not demonstrate the efficacy of either treatment. The investigator is limited to inferring, depending on the results, that one treatment is the same as, better than, or worse than the other. Thus, even though the trial is randomised, lack of control does not permit demonstration of Class I evidence.

THE DATA

Using the above definitions of the treatment outcome research terminology, the five-phase outcomes research model, and a level of evidence scale permits evaluation of the computerised aphasia treatment research literature. Discussion of the following investigations is intended to illustrate the application of some "rules to live by" in evaluating computer-provided aphasia treatment outcome research, and is not a comprehensive review of the computerised aphasia treatment outcome research literature. Eight Phase 1 studies, three series of Phase 2 studies, and a single Phase 3 study are considered.

Phase 1 studies

Seron, Deloche, Moulard, and Rouselle (1980) described a computer/clinician combination designed to help patients with aphasia learn to type and write a total of 90 words to dictation. The participants attempted to type a word on the computer keyboard after hearing the word spoken by the clinician. Only correctly typed letters were shown on the screen; errors were never displayed (and thus not "reinforced") by the computer. Intervention consisted of three levels of feedback: the number of letters in the target word (indicated by blank lines); whether the letter typed was in the word (indicated by displaying the letter somewhere on the screen); and when the correct letter was typed, whether that letter was in the correct position (indicated by displaying the letter in the correct position). Five participants, at least 3 months post-onset and representing a variety of aetiologies, completed the program in 7–30 sessions. To assess generalisation to writing, participants wrote a list of 50 words to dictation before beginning intervention and upon completion of the computer program. A decrease ($p < .05$) in the number of misspelled words and in the total number of errors made on the first post-treatment measure for the group of five participants supported the hypothesis that practice using the computer program may be active in improving writing words to dictation. Four of the five participants maintained improved performance on a second post-treatment test administered 6 weeks following termination of treatment. This constitutes a Phase I study and provides Class III evidence.

Mills (1982) reported using computer-controlled digitised speech to provide one-, two-, and three-step auditory "pointing" commands out of a field of four pictures in a simple drill for a patient with global aphasia at 16 months post-onset. Intervention was limited to repetitions of the auditory stimulus. After 13 months of treatment, improvement was described on post-treatment testing with the Porch Index of Communicative Ability (PICA) (Porch, 1981) auditory comprehension subtests VI (+4.8 points) and X (+1.5 points) and on an unspecified version of the Token Test (+23 percentile points). This Phase I study provides Class III evidence and suggests that the computer treatment was active.

Katz and Nagy (1982) described a computer program designed to test changes in reading comprehension and to provide reading stimulation for five patients with aphasia. The program consisted of 10 assessment subtests and six treatment tasks. Participants responded by pressing single keys to indicate choices. Feedback was limited to accuracy of response and was not corrective (Schuell et al., 1964). The people with aphasia ran the computer programs two to four times each week for 8 to 12 weeks with minimal assistance from the experimenters. Several participants demonstrated improved accuracy, decreased response latency, and increased the number of completed items on some computer tasks, but improvement in pre- to post-treatment test performance was minimal. This Phase 1 study suggests that while independent use of a computer to provide treatment was feasible for some patients with aphasia, the intervention did not indicate that the treatment was active.

Katz and Nagy (1983) reported a drill and practice (match-to-sample) computer program that was intended to improve visual word recognition for five chronic aphasic patients. The program presented 65 commonly occurring words. The word stimuli were randomly presented four times during each session. A complex, branching algorithm varied the duration of (tachistoscopic) exposure of each word as a function of the accuracy of prior responses. The goal of the program was to help increase and stabilise the patients' "sight vocabulary". This Phase 1, non-linguistic intervention (i.e., duration of exposure) did not appear to be active, because no improvement was observed when pre- and post-treatment measures were compared.

Scott and Byng (1989) tested the effectiveness of a computer program designed to improve comprehension of homophones for a subject who suffered traumatic head injury and underwent subsequent left temporal lobe surgery. Eight months after the accident, the subject continued to demonstrate aphasic symptoms as well as surface dyslexia and surface dysgraphia. Her reading was slow and laboured; however she was able to understand printed words by sounding them out. However, she demonstrated specific problems with homophones. The computer program, based on an information-processing model, was designed to focus on the homophone aspect of her reading problem. She demonstrated steady improvement on the 136-item treatment program, which was run 29 times over a 10-week period. The patient improved in her recognition and comprehension of treated (p < .001) and untreated (p < .002) homophones presented in sentences. Improvement was also demonstrated on recognition of isolated homophones that were treated (p < .05) and on defining isolated treated (p < .03) and untreated homophones (p < .02). Recognition of some untreated homophones and spelling of irregular words showed no improvement. Nevertheless, this Phase 1 study permits inference that the treatment was active and provides Level III evidence.

Deloche, Dordain, and Kremin (1993) developed software to treat oral and written modality differences in confrontation naming for two subjects with aphasia, one demonstrating surface dysgraphia (10 months post-onset) and the other demonstrating conduction aphasia (12 years post-onset). Each participant received 25 treatment sessions over six weeks. Intervention focused on typed naming responses, using the computer keyboard, following semantic and/or morpholexical (e.g., first letter, anagram) cues. Both participants showed improvement immediately following treatment as well as maintained improvement at 1 year after treatment. This Phase 1 study suggests that the treatment was active and provides Class III evidence.

Crerar and Ellis (1995) and Crerar, Ellis, and Dean (1996) described a computer system to treat sentence processing (comprehension) impairments, based on neuro-psychologic and psycholinguistic theory, in patients with chronic Broca's aphasia. A cross-over design was used to compare the performance of two groups of seven participants. One group received treatment on verbs followed by prepositions. The order was reversed (prepositions followed by verbs) for the second group. Graphic representations of agent, action, object, and spatial relations concepts were manipulated. Treatment was provided for 2 hours each week for 3 weeks. The authors reported that while the majority of patients obtained higher scores on verb and preposition tests, only three subjects showed statistically significant improvement. Follow-up evaluation after 5 months (during which no treatment was provided) indicated no differences between the groups or between treated and untreated items. This Phase 1 study provides mixed results. The treatment appeared to be active for some, but not all, participants.

The above Phase 1 studies provide mixed results. In some, the treatment provided appeared to be active, as demonstrated by improved pre- to post-treatment performance on the outcome measures employed. The level of evidence provided in the studies that reported improvement is Class III, because all utilised a single small group or a case report. In studies where the treatment appeared to be active, the investigators were justified in initiating Phase 2 research.

Phase 2 studies

Three series of studies are described to demonstrate the progression of Phase 1 research in Phase 2 investigations. Utilising the results of Phase 1 research, the investigators proceeded programmatically to achieve some of the purposes of Phase 2 research described above.

Katz and colleagues reported three studies designed to approximate the decision-making process of a clinician by providing hierarchically arranged cues. Each new treatment session began at the level completed at the end of the last session. In addition, printed, performance-specific homework was provided. Building on earlier, Phase 1 studies (Katz & Nagy, 1982, 1983; Seron et al., 1980), Katz and Nagy (1984) incorporated complex branching steps in a computer program to evaluate aphasic patients' responses and to provide them with error-specific, linguistically relevant feedback in a computerised, typing/handwriting, confrontation naming/spelling task. A stimulus word was randomly selected from a pool of 10 by the program, and a drawing representing the word was displayed on the computer screen. Participants responded by typing letters on the keyboard. Feedback consisted of auditory tones (indicating correct and incorrect responses), and text messages were printed on the screen. Single and multiple cues, from a hierarchy of six, were selected by the program in response to the number of errors made. Specific cues included anagrams, multiple-choices, copying from a model, and modelling from memory. A 7-point scoring system was used to describe performance and track the influence of each cue. Additional feedback included repetition of the successful stimuli and the most recently successful cues. At the end of each computer session, performance-specific, pencil-and-paper copying assignments were automatically generated by the computer printer as homework to be completed by each participant. Comparison of pre- and post-writing tests revealed improved spelling of the target words for seven of the eight aphasic participants ($p < .01$). This Phase II study, building on previous Phase 1 research, provides Class III evidence and demonstrates that the intervention (treatment hierarchy and copying assignment) was active.

Katz and Nagy (1985) used a similar algorithm to create a self-modifying drill and practice (match-to-sample) program designed to improve reading comprehension, without clinician assistance, for 12 common words (e.g., spoon, fork, etc.) for adults with aphasia. Participants were asked to "find the word that is the name of the picture" from among two to six multiple choice alternatives. Beginning with two alternatives, the number of choices and the complexity of foils (from visually to semantically confusing) increased as a result of the participant's previous accurate responses. Subsequent sessions automatically began at the level last completed, as in typical, clinician-provided treatment, rather than starting at the lowest level of the treatment hierarchy, as in most computer programs. The program also generated, through a printer, homework (writing activities) that corresponded to each participant's performance. The five aphasic participants ranged in pre- to post-treatment improvement (percent correct) on the treatment items from 0% to 54%, with an average of 26.6% ($p < .05$). This Phase 2 study provides Level III evidence that the treatment was active for some participants with aphasia. A natural progression would be additional Phase 2 research designed to demonstrate selection criteria to determine which people with aphasia would benefit from the treatment.

Katz, Wertz, Davidoff, Schubitowski, and Devitt (1989) developed and tested a computer program for aphasic patients designed to improve written confrontation naming of animals. As in previous Phase 1 research, the program was designed to require no assistance from a clinician. The treatment program required subjects to type the names of 10 animals in response to pictures displayed on the computer monitor. If the name was typed correctly, feedback was provided, and another picture was displayed. If an error was made, hierarchically arranged cues were presented, and response requirements were modified. Nine participants with aphasia improved from pre- to post-treatment an average of 40% on the computer task ($p < .0001$). Five participants reached criterion performance within six treatment sessions. Generalisation to handwriting was demonstrated for written confrontation naming of the treatment stimuli and written generative naming (word fluency) for animal names ($p < .001$). Improvement did not, nor was it expected to, generalise to written word fluency for an unrelated category. In addition, the groups' PICA Writing modality score improved by +4.1 percentile points ($p < .05$). However, results did not generalise to significant improvement in PICA Overall and Reading scores. This Phase 2 study demonstrated that the computer-provided treatment, without clinician assistance, was active, and it provides Level III evidence.

Loverso and colleagues conducted three computerised/clinician-assisted studies (Loverso, Prescott, Selinger, & Riley, 1988; Loverso, Prescott, & Selinger, 1992; Loverso, Prescott, Selinger, Wheeler, & Smith, 1985), based on Phase 1 research that developed and explored a model-driven, clinician-provided treatment approach, the "verb as core" (Loverso, Prescott, & Selinger, 1988; Loverso, Selinger, & Prescott., 1979). Verbs were presented as starting points and paired with different wh-question words to provide cues designed to elicit sentences in an actor-action-object framework from participants with aphasia. Thirty verbs were used in each of six modules. A hierarchy was divided into two major levels, each consisting of an initial module and two sub-modules that provided additional cueing for participants with aphasia who were unable to achieve 60% or better accuracy on the initial module. Level I presented stimulus verbs and the question words "who" or "what" to elicit an actor-action sentence. Level II elicited actor-action-object sentences by presenting stimulus verbs and the question words "who" or "what" for the actor and the question words "how", "when", "where", and "why" for the object. Participants responded verbally and graphically. The treatment was provided three to five times per week. During each session, 30 stimulus verbs were presented for generation of sentences. An alternating treatment design with multiple internal (i.e., generalisation set of stimulus items) and external (i.e., PICA testing pre- and post-treatment) probes was utilised. A no-treatment control group was not employed. Statistically significant improvement ($p < .05$) was demonstrated on the PICA following 3.5 months of treatment for each of two participants with aphasia.

Loverso et al. (1985) compared the effects of verbing treatment provided by a clinician with similar treatment provided by a computer and speech synthesiser and assistance by a clinician. A participant with aphasia responded in the clinician-only condition by speaking and writing, and in the clinician/computer condition by speaking and typing. Stimulus presentation and feedback in the clinician/computer condition were provided only by the computer. The clinician intervened only if the participant's typed response was correct but the spoken response was in error. The same single-subject design used in Loverso et al. (1979) was employed. The participant improved on the task under both conditions but took longer to reach criterion performance in the computer and clinician-assisted condition. Based on the participant's improvement, both on the treatment task and on "clinically meaningful" changes on successive administrations of the PICA ($p < .01$), the authors concluded that their listening, reading, and typing activities had a positive influence on the aphasic participant's language performance.

Loverso et al. (1988) expanded on Loverso et al. (1985) by comparing the performance of subjects with fluent and nonfluent aphasia. Subjects in both groups required an average of 28% more sessions ($p < .05$) to reach criterion performance in the computer/clinician condition than in the clinician-only condition. Fluent subjects required 24% more sessions, and non-fluent subjects required 33% more sessions. Eight subjects showed significant improvement ($p < .05$) post-treatment on PICA Overall, Verbal modality, and Graphic modality scores. All of these subjects maintained their gains after 1 month post-treatment. Loverso et al. (1992) replicated the study with 20 subjects with aphasia and reported similar results. These Phase 2 studies indicate that the treatment was active for some people with aphasia, and they provide Class III evidence.

Steele, Weinrich, and their colleagues measured the effect of a non-verbal, language-like computerised symbolic communication system on adults with aphasia. Their work was based on work designed to teach non-human primates (e.g., chimpanzees, apes) to use non-verbal, language-like (non-computerised) symbolic communication systems (Gardner and Gardner, 1969; Premack, 1970). These efforts led to the application of the approach with severely aphasic people (e.g., Gardner, Zurif, Berry, & Baker, 1976). Developing the concept further, Steele, Weinrich, Kleczewska, Wertz, and Carlson (1987) and Steele, Weinrich, Wertz, Kleczewska, and Carlson (1989) developed a graphically oriented, computer-based, alternative communication system called the Computerized Visual Communication system (C-VIC) for chronic, globally aphasic adults. C-VIC employed an interactive pointing board that ran on a Macintosh computer and used a picture-card design, similar to the "folder" concept used on computer desktops. Participants with aphasia used the mouse to select one of several icons, each of which represented a distinct category (e.g., things, actions, modifiers, etc.). The selected icon then "opened" to reveal pictures of subfolders or items within the category. After selecting the desired item, the picture was added to a sequence of other selected pictures, and this "string" of pictures represented the message. The message could be read as the sequence of icons; words printed below the sequence; or, in some cases, heard as digitised speech.

The empirical evidence to support the use of C-VIC was collected in a series of single-case studies (Weinrich, McCall, Shoosmith, Thomas, Katzenberger, & Weber, 1993; Weinrich, Steele, Kleczewska, Carlson, Baker, & Wertz, 1989). Steele et al. (1987) reported that, although globally impaired aphasic participants could employ C-VIC to improve their expressive and receptive performance, communication in more traditional modes—speaking, writing, reading, auditory comprehension—remained unchanged. Thus, while C-VIC training improved the aphasic participants' communicative ability, it did not generalise to improved performance in natural language.

A commercial version of C-VIC, called Lingraphica, was developed to incorporate animation and digitised speech on a Macintosh PowerBook computer. Lingraphica is an integrated, computerised communication system that combines spoken words, printed words, pictures (icons), and text processing. Aphasic patients use a mouse device to select one of several icons each representing a general category. The selected icon then "opens up" to reveal pictures of the items within the selected category. After selecting the desired item, the picture is added to a sequence of other selected pictures, and this "string" of pictures represents the message, which can be read as the sequence of icons, words printed below the sequence, or heard through digitised speech. Aftonomos, Steele, and Wertz (1997) used Lingraphica with 20 participants with aphasia and reported improvement in natural language in multiple modalities for most participants, including oral-expressive language. The treatment approach reported by Aftonomos et al. (1997) formed the basis of a multi-modal treatment for aphasia administered by speech-language pathologists using Lingraphica in LingraphiCare clinics. Thus, building on the early C-VIC Phase 1 research, the LingraphiCare treatment reported in Phase 2 research is designed to improve performance in natural language. The Aftonomos et al. (1997) results imply the treatment is active and provides Class III evidence.

Phase III studies

To our knowledge, there has been only one Phase 3 investigation designed to test the efficacy of computer-provided treatment for aphasia. Katz and Wertz (1997) conducted a longitudinal, group study to investigate the effects of computerised language activities and computer stimulation on language improvement in chronic aphasic adults. A total of 55 chronic aphasic participants who were no longer receiving speech-language therapy were assigned randomly to one of three conditions: 78 hours of computer reading treatment, 78 hours of computer stimulation ("non-language" activities), or no-treatment. The computer reading treatment software consisted of 29 activities, each containing eight levels of difficulty, that comprised a total of 232 different tasks. Treatment tasks required visual-matching and reading comprehension skills, displayed only text (no pictures), and used a standard, match-to-sample format with two to five multiple choices. Treatment incorporated principles of Schuell's (1974) stimulation approach in which patients are treated as active participants in the reorganisation of language. The treatment was designed to maximise interaction (Duffy & Coelho, 2001) so that participants with aphasia responded frequently and, usually, accurately, while still finding the task challenging. Treatment software automatically adjusted task difficulty, in response to participant performance, by incorporating traditional treatment procedures, for example, hierarchically arranged tasks and measurement of performance on baseline and generalisation stimulus sets, in conjunction with complex branching algorithms. Software used in the computer stimulation condition was a combination of cognitive rehabilitation software and computer games that used movement, shape, and/or colour to focus on reaction time, attention span, memory, and other skills that did not overtly require language or other communication abilities. The purpose of the computer stimulation condition was to determine whether improvement from pre- to post-treatment on language outcome measures resulted from the language stimuli present in the computer reading treatment, or whether improvement resulted simply from the stimulation provided by using a computer in the stimulation condition. Subjects in the two computer conditions used the computer for 3 hours each week for 26 weeks. Clinician interaction during the two computer conditions was minimal. Participants in all three conditions were tested with the PICA and the Western Aphasia Battery (WAB) (Kertesz, 1982) at pre-treatment, after 3 months of treatment, and after 6 months of treatment. Significant pre- to post-treatment improvement over the 26-week treatment trial occurred on five language measures for the computer reading treatment group, on one language measure for the computer stimulation group, and on none of the language measures for the no-treatment group. The computer reading treatment group displayed significantly more improvement on the PICA Overall and Verbal modality percentiles and on the WAB Aphasia Quotient and Repetition subtest than the other two groups. The results suggest that: computerised reading treatment can be administered with minimal assistance from a clinician; improvement on the computerised reading treatment tasks generalised to non-computer language performance; improvement resulted from the language content of the software and not simply stimulation provided by a computer; and the computerised reading treatment provided to chronic aphasic patients was efficacious.

The Katz and Wertz (1997) investigation represents a computer-provided intervention for a specific language behaviour—reading. All participants with aphasia received the same treatment, and each participant was exposed to a systematic hierarchy of language-based treatment stimuli. The design tested the efficacy of what is considered a cognitive-linguistic remediation. The evidence for the treatment's efficacy is based on the time elapsed post-CVA—all participants demonstrated chronic aphasia—and, more importantly, demonstration of significantly more improvement in the randomly assigned computer reading treatment group than in the randomly assigned computer stimulation and no-treatment groups. This Phase 3 study provided Class 1 evidence, with results from a well-designed, randomised controlled clinical trial that compared treatment with no-treatment.

Phase 4 and 5 studies

We know of no Phase 4 or 5 studies in the computer-provided aphasia treatment literature. Using the treatment outcome research rule that Phase 4 and 5 effectiveness and efficiency studies are conducted only after demonstrating a treatment's efficacy in Phase 3, only the Katz and Wertz (1997) computer reading treatment would qualify for testing in Phase 4 and 5 effectiveness research.

CONCLUSIONS

The available support to justify computer-provided treatment for people with aphasia is, primarily, Class III evidence, expert opinion, non-randomised historical controls, or one or more case reports, obtained in the Phase 1 and 2 investigations reviewed above. Only one investigation (Katz & Wertz, 1997) provides Class I evidence. Certainly, there is work to be done.

We suggest that future investigations be guided by the "rules to live by" provided by Robey and Schultz (1998): precise definitions of the treatment outcomes research terminology; programmatic development of a treatment by meeting the purposes of each phase in the five-phase treatment outcomes research model; and application of a Level of Evidence Scale to rate the results provided by each investigation in each phase of the model. Moreover, continued research on computer-provided treatment for aphasia should consider Robey's (1998, p. 183) observation and suggestions for treatment outcome research on aphasia in general:

> Many studies have treated omnibus hypotheses (e.g., heterogeneous patients improve with the administration of heterogeneous treatments provided on heterogeneous schedules in heterogeneous contexts; ... focused hypotheses must be tested programmatically (e.g., replications on tests of dosage, specific populations, certain severities, and treatment protocols...

Aphasiologists should not expect computer-provided treatment to be efficacious simply because it is based on clinician-provided efficacious treatment. The introduction of computers in the rehabilitation of language and communication for people with aphasia has renewed recognition of treatment as a multifaceted, behaviour exchange. Clinicians cannot anticipate all possible patient behaviours, and developers of computer-provided treatment programs can only code a limited number of contingencies. As long as computer treatment programs are based on convergent, rather than divergent, theories of learning, computerised treatment will remain a subset of clinician-provided treatment. While computers may function faster than clinicians and, perhaps, be able to provide an increased dosage (amount of stimulation-facilitation), treatment provided by a computer may remain a supplement to treatment provided by a clinician. This, however, is a testable hypothesis. Continued Phase 1–5 computer-provided treatment for aphasia will provide the empirical evidence for acceptance or rejection of the hypothesis. As always, over the mountains are mountains.

REFERENCES

Aftonomos, L. B., Steele, R. D., & Wertz, R. T. (1997). Promoting recovery in chronic aphasia with an interactive technology. *Archives of Physical Medicine, 78,* 841–846.

American Academy of Neurology Therapeutics and Technology Assessment Subcommittee (1994). Assessment: Melodic intonation therapy. *Neurology, 44,* 566–568.

Crerar, M. A., & Ellis, A. W. (1995). Computer-based therapy for aphasia: Towards second generation clinical tools. In C. Code & D. Müller (Eds.), *Treatment of aphasia: From theory to practice* (pp. 223–250). London: Whurr Publishers Ltd.

Crerar, M. A., Ellis, A. W., & Dean, E. C. (1996). Remediation of sentence processing deficits in aphasia using a computer-based microworld. *Brain and Language, 52,* 229–275.

Deloche, G., Dordain, M., & Kremin, H. (1993). Rehabilitation of confrontational naming in aphasia: Relations between oral and written modalities. *Aphasiology, 7,* 201–216.

Duffy, J. R., & Coelho, C. A. (2001). Schuell's stimulation approach to rehabilitation. In R. Chapey (Ed.), *Language intervention strategies in aphasia and related neurogenic communication disorders* (4th ed.) (pp. 341–382). Philadelphia: Lippincott Williams & Wilkins.

Gardner, H., Zurif, E., Berry, T., & Baker, E. (1976). Visual communication in aphasia. *Neuropsychologia, 14,* 275–292.

Gardner, R., & Gardner, B. (1969). Teaching sign language to a chimpanzee. *Science, 165,* 664–672.

Horner, J., Loverso, F. L., & Gonzalez Rothi, L. (1994). Models of aphasia treatment. In R. Chapey (Ed.), *Language intervention strategies in adult aphasia* (4th ed.) (pp. 1135–1145). Baltimore: Williams & Wilkins.

Katz, R. C., & Nagy, V. T. (1982). A computerized treatment system for chronic aphasic adults. In R. H. Brookshire (Ed.), *Clinical aphasiology: 1982 conference proceedings* (pp. 153–160). Minneapolis, MN: BRK Publishers.

Katz, R. C., & Nagy, V. T. (1983). A computerized approach for improving word recognition in chronic aphasic patients. In R. H. Brookshire (Ed.), *Clinical aphasiology: 1983 conference proceedings* (pp. 65–72). Minneapolis, MN: BRK Publishers.

Katz, R. C., & Nagy, V. T. (1984). An intelligent computer-based task for chronic aphasic patients. In R. H. Brookshire (Ed.), *Clinical aphasiology: 1984 conference proceedings* (pp. 159–165). Minneapolis, MN: BRK Publishers.

Katz, R. C., & Nagy, V. T. (1985). A self-modifying computerized reading program for severely-impaired aphasic adults. In R. H. Brookshire (Ed.), *Clinical aphasiology: 1985 conference proceedings* (pp. 184–188). Minneapolis, MN: BRK Publishers.

Katz, R. C., & Wertz, R. T. (1997). The efficacy of computer-provided reading treatment for chronic aphasic adults. *Journal of Speech, Language and Hearing Research, 40,* 493–507.

Katz, R. C., Wertz, R. T., Davidoff, M., Schubitowski, Y. D., &. Devitt, E. W. (1989). A computer program to improve written confrontation naming in aphasia. In T. E. Prescott (Ed.), *Clinical aphasiology: 1988 conference proceedings* (pp. 321–338), Austin, TX: Pro-Ed.

Kertesz, A. (1982). *Western aphasia battery.* New York: Grune & Stratton.

Loverso, F. L., Prescott, T. E., & Selinger, M. (1988). Cueing verbs: A treatment strategy for aphasic adults. *Journal of Rehabilitation Research and Development, 25,* 47–60.

Loverso, F. L., Prescott, T. E., & Selinger, M. (1992). Microcomputer treatment applications in aphasiology. *Aphasiology, 6,* 155–163.

Loverso, F. L., Prescott, T. E., Selinger, M., & Riley, L. (1988). Comparison of two modes of aphasia treatment: Clinician and computer-clinician assisted. In T. E. Prescott (Ed.), *Clinical aphasiology* (Vol. 18, pp. 297–319). Austin, TX: Pro-Ed.

Loverso, F. L., Prescott, T. E., Selinger, M., Wheeler, K. M., & Smith, R. D. (1985). The application of microcomputers for the treatment of aphasic adults. In R. H. Brookshire (Ed.), *Clinical aphasiology: 1985 conference proceedings* (pp. 189–195). Minneapolis, MN: BRK Publishers.

Loverso, F. L., Selinger, M., & Prescott, T. E. (1979). Application of verbing strategies to aphasia treatment. In R. H. Brookshire (Ed.), *Clinical aphasiology: 1979 conference proceedings* (pp. 229–238). Minneapolis, MN: BRK Publishers.

Mills, R. H. (1982). Microcomputerized auditory comprehension training. In R. H. Brookshire (Ed.), *Clinical aphasiology: 1982 conference proceedings* (pp. 147–152). Minneapolis, MN: BRK Publishers.

Office of Technology Assessment (1978). *Assessing the efficacy and safety of medical technologies. OTA-H-75.* Washington, DC: US Government Printing Office.

Porch, B. E. (1981). *Porch Index of Communicative Ability, Vol. 1: Administration, scoring, and interpretation* (3rd ed.). Palo Alto, CA: Consulting Psychologists Press.

Premack, D. (1970). The education of Sarah: A chimp learns the language. *Psychology Today, 4,* 55–58.

Robey, R. R. (1998). A meta-analysis of clinical outcomes in the treatment of aphasia. *Journal of Speech, Language, and Hearing Research, 41,* 172–187.

Robey, R. R., & Schultz, M. C. (1998). A model for conducting clinical-outcome research: An adaptation of the standard protocol for use in aphasiology. *Aphasiology, 12,* 787–810.

Robinson, I. (1990). Does computerized cognitive rehabilitation work? *Aphasiology, 4,* 381–405.

Schuell, H. (1974). *Aphasia theory and therapy: Selected lectures and papers of Hildred* Schuell. Baltimore: Park Press.

Schuell, H., Jenkins, J. J., & Jiménez-Pabón, E. (1964). *Aphasia in adults.* New York: Harper & Row.

Scott, C., & Byng, S. (1989). Computer-assisted remediation of a homophone comprehension disorder in surface dyslexia. *Aphasiology, 3,* 301–320.

Sederer, L. I., Dickey, B., & Hermann, R. C. (1996). The imperative of outcomes assessment in psychiatry. In L. I. Sederer & B. Dickey (Eds.), *Outcomes assessment in clinical practice* (pp. 1–7). Baltimore: Williams & Wilkins.

Seron, X., Deloche, G., Moulard, G., & Rouselle, M. (1980). A computer-based therapy for the treatment of aphasic subjects with writing disorders. *Journal of Speech and Hearing Disorders, 45,* 45–58.

Steele, R. D., Weinrich, M., Kleczewska, M. K., Wertz, R. T., & Carlson, G. S. (1987). Evaluating performance of severely aphasic patients on a computer-aided visual communication system. In R. H. Brookshire (Ed.), *Clinical aphasiology: 1987 conference proceedings* (pp. 46–54). Minneapolis, MN: BRK Publishers.

Steele, R. D., Weinrich, M., Wertz, R. T., Kleczewska, M. K., & Carlson, G. S. (1989). Computer-based visual communication in aphasia. *Neuropsychologia, 27,* 409–427.

Weinrich, M., McCall, D., Shoosmith, L., Thomas, K., Katzenberger, K., & Weber, C. (1993). Locative prepositional phrases in severe aphasia. *Brain and Language, 45,* 21–45.

Weinrich, M., Steele, R. D., Kleczewska, M., Carlson, G. S., Baker, E., & Wertz, R. T. (1989). Representation of "verbs" in a computerized visual communication system. *Aphasiology, 3*(6), 501–512.

Wertz, R. T., & Irwin, W. H. (2001). Darley and the efficacy of language rehabilitation in aphasia. *Aphasiology, 15,* 231–247.

APHASIOLOGY, 2004, *18* (3), 245–263

High-tech AAC and aphasia: Widening horizons?

Mieke W. M. E. van de Sandt-Koenderman

Rijndam Rehabilitation Centre/Rotterdam Aphasia Foundation, The Netherlands

Background: Many people with aphasia are trained to use low-tech AAC strategies (Alternative and Augmentative Communication) to support communication, but high-tech communication aids are introduced only incidentally. The factors influencing success and failure of low-tech AAC are relevant for the development of high-tech communication aids for aphasia.

Aims: To review the state of the art in low-tech and high-tech AAC applications for aphasia.

Main Contribution: Although there is there is a wealth of knowledge among therapists, there is very little research to support the efficacy of AAC techniques. Many authors stress the heterogeneity of the aphasic population, not only in the characteristics of the aphasia, but also in communicative abilities and needs, cognitive abilities, motivation, and social situation. Therefore, AAC devices should be individualised and "tailor-made", taking advantage of residual language skills and communicative strengths. A common problem is that acquired AAC skills are often not used in daily communication. Several factors may play a role, e.g., lack of motivation, inadequate vocabulary, insufficient training, or cognitive or linguistic limitations. So far, functional use of assistive technology has received relatively little attention, but a portable device with ready-made messages for specific communicative situations appeared to be used in every day life.

Conclusions: Computer technology has much to offer for supporting aphasic communication, not only for people with a very severe aphasia, who do not benefit from disorder-oriented therapy, but also for people with a moderate or mild aphasia. Research into AAC and aphasia, focusing on functional use, is needed in order to build and refine communication aids that are easy to use and can be tailored individually.

Since the introduction of the personal computer in the late 1970s, we have seen a rapid growth of computer technology. Computers have become faster and more reliable and also much smaller, with an enormous memory capacity and with multimedia applications. For most people the computer has become a necessary tool, both professionally and at home. The technology is still developing very fast, and a new computer will be outdated within one or two years.

Address correspondence to: Mieke W.M.E. van de Sandt,-Koenderman Rijndam Rehabilitation Centre/SAR, Westersingel 300, 3015 LJ Rotterdam, The Netherlands. Email: m.sandt@rijndam.nl

This review is partly based on the work done by the clinical partners of the PCAD project team (Telematics Application for Disabled and Elderly; TIDE 3211), P. Hardy, A. Davies, S. Woodward, J. Mortley, & P. Enderby (Speech and Language Therapy Research Unit, Bristol, UK), A. Lysley & R. Moore (ACE centre, Oxford, UK), F. Stachowiak & C. Wahn (University of Leipzig, Germany), A. Matos & B. Largo (Hospitais da Universidade de Coimbra, Portugal), P. Kitzing, (University of Lund, Sweden), and C. Kornman, J. Wiegers, & S. Wielaert (Rotterdam Aphasia Foundation, the Netherlands). I am very grateful to them for sharing their knowledge and their clinical experience. I also thank the technical partners P. Tippell & S. Whitehouse (Thames Valley University, London, UK), for their hard work in developing the Touch Speak software.

In this context, the development of computer applications for aphasia treatment seems to be rather slow and this especially holds true for the development of high-tech Alternative and Augmentative Communication (AAC) for people with aphasia. While during the 1980s and 1990s specific treatment software became available for aphasia therapy (e.g., Aftonomos, Steele, & Wertz, 1997; Katz, 2001; Katz & Wertz, 1997; Pedersen, Vinter & Olsen, 2001; Scott & Byng, 1989; Stachowiak, 1993; Stumpel, van Dijk, Messing-Peterson, & de Vries, 1989; van de Sandt-Koenderman & Visch-Brink, 1993; van Mourik & van de Sandt-Koenderman, 1992), the use of computer technology to support aphasic persons in their communication is restricted and has been developing at a slow pace.

Over a decade ago, Kraat stated that so far very few aphasic people with aphasias had benefited from AAC applications, but she expected "to see a proliferation of glittering technologies" offering unique options for functional AAC devices (Kraat, 1990, p. 334). Until now, however, the technological options have hardly been used to develop a whole generation of functional AAC devices for aphasic persons. In order to use the technological options available, cooperation between technicians and aphasiologists is required, and it is up to the clinicians to formulate the user requirements of the systems to be developed. Unfortunately however, aphasia specialists have limited knowledge of the state of the art in the field of high-tech AAC devices for other communicatively impaired groups; but even worse: many of them also have restricted views of what even low-tech AAC may contribute (Hux, Beukelman, & Garrett, 1994). To be able to develop communication aids, the lessons learnt from applying low-tech AAC strategies are crucial (Kraat, 1990). Another source of information is the use of AAC by people with other types of communicative disorders. This article will review the state of the art, both in low-tech and in high-tech AAC applications for aphasia. The review is partly based on the work of the international team that developed PCAD/Touchspeak (Personal Communication Assistant for Dysphasic People, commercially available as Touchspeak) and reflects the perspective of the clinical partners in the UK, Portugal, Germany, Sweden, and the Netherlands.

LOW-TECH AAC INTERVENTION IN APHASIA: WHAT ARE THE LESSONS?

The World Health Organisation (WHO, 2001) advocates shifting attention from the level of impairment to the levels of activities and participation. In the field of aphasia rehabilitation, this means that concepts like functional communication and communicative roles are now becoming more and more important for clinicians and researchers. Recent publications show the increased focus on the levels of activities and participation (e.g., Cruice, Worrall, Hickson, & Murison, 2003; Davidson, Worrall, & Hickson, 2003).

AAC training is an intervention at these levels and the field of AAC for aphasia is relatively young. The tradition of disorder-oriented language therapy goes back much further, usually focusing on auditory comprehension and spoken language production. For a long time, impairment-oriented treatment was seen as the best approach to achieve a higher level of communication. AAC strategies were often felt to be a last resort, to fall back on only if the restoration of language functions failed.

Compared to the extensive literature on impairment-oriented therapies, the literature on AAC strategies is limited. As a result, we know much more about the effect of therapy at the level of the language impairment than about the effect of training AAC strategies.

There is growing evidence that this approach is efficacious (Cicerone et al., 2000; Robey, 1994; Robey & Schultz, 1998; Whurr, Lorch, & Nye, 1992, 2000).

In contrast with these results, there are no Class I or Class II studies providing information about the effects of the application of AAC strategies in aphasia. The lessons that can be learned from the application of low-tech AAC strategies so far are mainly based on case studies and on the expertise of experienced clinicians all over the world.

LOW-TECH AAC STRATEGIES

To support the communication of people with severe aphasia, several other channels can be used to get the message across, either verbal (writing, alphabet board, choice from written words/messages) or nonverbal (gestures, mimic, drawing, pictures, symbols, photographs) (Hux, Manasse, Weiss, & Beukelman, 2001).

Writing

Spoken and written output may be differentially impaired. For example, persons with a severe apraxia of speech may only have a mild form of aphasia; in other people, there may be a dissociation between the phonological output route and the graphemic output route (Hier & Mohr, 1977; Semenza, Cippolotti, & Denes, 1992; Visch-Brink, 1999). Both types of patients have relatively good writing skills, but are unable to speak. For those patients who are able to produce (part of the) written word form instead of the spoken word form, writing may contribute to their communication. Even for people with limited skills, writing may be beneficial, because the first letters of a word may provide the communication partner with a basis for "intelligent guessing". When writing is impossible due to motor problems, an alphabet board might be used to point to relevant letters.

The non-aphasic communication partner may also use writing to support language comprehension. People with severe aphasia often find it easier to understand when the message is given in two input modalities in parallel. Written choice communication, where the communication partner offers written alternatives, can be a very useful AAC technique to support conversation (Garrett & Beukelman, 1992; Verschaeve & Wielaert, 1994).

Gestures, mimicking, pointing

Some patients are very proficient in using nonverbal channels like gesturing, mimicking, and pointing. Many people with severe aphasia also suffer from limb apraxia and their ability to produce gestures may be restricted. However, Feyereisen, Barter, Goossens, and Clerebaut (1988) studied comprehension and production of gestures in a group of 12 people with aphasia and found that limb apraxia was negatively correlated with the use of gestures: more gestures were used by the people with more severe apraxia.

Natural gestures provide a limited channel: gestures are often ambiguous, and can only refer to a reduced set of—mainly concrete—concepts. Often the gestures are only comprehensible in the situational context (Feyereisen et al., 1988). It is easy to use a gesture to ask for the hammer when standing next to a toolbox, but it is difficult to refer to the fact that you have been a biotechnologist, or that you worry about your daughter's health.

A formal system of gestures (e.g., AmerInd; Rao, 2001) can only be used with a restricted number of communication partners, since it is necessary that the communication partners are able to comprehend the sign language.

Drawing

The aphasic person may use communicative drawing to convey his/her messages (Lyon, 1995). For many people drawing will be a communication mode that does not come naturally, but has to be trained in aphasia therapy. Like writing, drawing may also be used by the communication partner to support the person with aphasia's language comprehension.

Drawing skills vary considerably, also in non-aphasic communicators. In the aphasic population constructional disorders may occur as a result of the brain damage causing the aphasia. These may prevent the person with aphasia from using drawing as a mode for communication.

Communication books

Communication books and communication boards can be used to point to words, pictures, photographs or symbols. Generic communication books have a fixed vocabulary and can be used to express wants and needs, and to answer questions. During therapy the person with aphasia has to learn to find specific items.

The organisation of the vocabulary is an important factor. The vocabulary organisation of non-aphasic speakers is largely unknown and it is possible that the organisation chosen for AAC systems is artificial and not easy to learn. Two Dutch communication books that are used very frequently for persons with a severe aphasia differ in organisation. The Taalzakboek ("Language Pocket Book") provides a vocabulary of pictures and words, organised in semantic categories like bathroom, food, professions, traffic etc. (de Vries, Stumpel, Stoutjesdijk, & Barf, 2001). The *Gespreksboek* ("Conversation Book") is organised around speech acts (telling, asking, requests) and around the key questions: "who", "what", and "where" (Verschaeve & Wielaert, 1994). Clinicians tend to use the *Taalzakboek* for the more severe patients, assuming that the organisation in categories is easier for persons with a very severe aphasia.

For patients who have limited skills in using a communication book, it may be used by the healthy partner to ask questions and provide a choice of words/pictures as possible answers. No evaluation studies of the use of communication books have been published, and no selection criteria are known so far. Possibly, those patients with relatively good reading and cognitive skills will be able to use a book system independently to convey their messages and to initiate communication.

In practice, some people with aphasia, especially in the first year post onset, refuse to learn to use a communication book, either because they don't accept the fact that they might need a supportive system, or because they feel the book system does not meet their needs. When an person is able to use the book during therapy, this does not guarantee that it will be used functionally, in conversation with familiar or unfamiliar communication partners.

Personalised communication books are sometimes extensions of generic communication books, with extra sections for personal information, e.g., names of family members, personal history, favourite sport clubs etc. The book may also provide a page with instructions for communication partners: a description of AAC techniques that the person with aphasia finds helpful, e.g., it may ask the listener to speak slowly, or to support spoken messages with written words. These instructions may also be written on a communication card, which can be kept to hand in all situations (Garrett & Beukelman, 1992).

Garrett and Huth (2002) used "graphic topic setters" to support conversation. These tangible referents (e.g., Communication books, photographs, newspapers) served as conversational resources during interactions of a severely aphasic communicator with two non-aphasic conversation partners. The authors videotaped conversations with and without graphic topic setters. Analysis showed that graphic topic setters facilitated conversation.

FACTORS INFLUENCING SUCCESS OF LOW-TECH AAC

Aphasia

Several authors stress the heterogenic nature of the client group, even within the standard aphasia types (Garrett & Beukelman, 1992; Hux et al., 1994; Hux et al., 2001; Kraat, 1990; Shelton, Weinrich, McCall, & Cox, 1996). People with restricted verbal production show considerable variation in linguistic skills. For example, auditory comprehension may vary from severely disturbed to almost normal, and semantic processing varies to the same extent (Visch-Brink, 1999). An important factor is the possible dissociation between speaking and writing. For some people who can hardly speak, writing is much easier; in others, reading comprehension may be the best or the worst modality.

When planning an AAC intervention, it is important to use all client resources and to stress the person with aphasia's strengths, rather than weaknesses, to optimise communication (Garrett & Beukelman, 1992; Hux et al., 2001). Hence, type and severity of aphasia are insufficient indicators of how successful an aid might be, and AAC assessment asks for more than the administration of a standard aphasia battery.

Cognition

The person with aphasia, like other brain-damaged people, may experience slowing of thought, emotional instability, and reduced energy. Furthermore, severe aphasia often occurs in combination with other neuropsychological deficits as a result of the focal brain damage that caused the aphasia. There may be specific memory problems, hemi-inattention, acalculia, visuo-spatial problems, and/or a disturbance in the executive control functions (van Mourik, Verschaeve, Boon, Paquier, & van Harskamp, 1992; Visch-Brink, van Harskamp, van Amerongen, Wielaert, & van de Sandt-Koenderman, 1993). Assessing cognitive functions in this group is problematic due to the language disorder, since "language-free neuropsychological assessment" is only possible in a restricted way.

Although it is plausible that a certain level of cognitive functioning is a prerequisite for learning to use AAC techniques, there is no research available in this field. The role of cognition in the use of high-tech and low-tech AAC has so far been largely ignored (Light & Lindsay, 1991). It is not unlikely that cognitive problems (e.g. disturbance of initiative and/or executive control functions) are responsible for the lack of functional use of AAC in some clients. They are able to use a specific AAC system inside the therapy room, but do not use it functionally, in daily life.

Acceptance

The acceptance of AAC strategies and devices by people with aphasia and their communicative environment is problematic. Many clients, but possibly even more often their spouses, have problems with accepting AAC, because they feel that using AAC means giving up the hope of recovering natural speech.

Hux et al. (2001) stress that AAC techniques are used by non-communicatively disabled speakers as well. They will use gestures to support speech in a noisy room, or they will write down words a communication partner is not familiar with, or they will use a map when explaining a route somewhere. Therefore, "viewing AAC techniques as a natural part of communicative interactions—those generated by disabled and non-disabled speakers—eliminates some of the stigma associated with using substitutions for natural speech" (Hux et al., 2001, p. 681).

The expected role of AAC

Depending on the severity of the aphasia, a system may be used for replacing, supplementing, or scaffolding natural speech (Hux et al., 2001). It is often stressed that AAC should not be seen as a last resort for those patients who do not respond to therapy aimed at restoration of verbal communication. Some of the roles that have been suggested are: supplementing communication in a particular communicative situation, predicting what a person is saying from minimal input, accomplishing social interaction, increasing comprehension in Wernicke's aphasics and expanding one- or two-word utterances of Broca's patients into complete sentences (Kraat, 1990).

Most authors agree that no AAC system can replace natural communication. It should always have an augmentative role and people with aphasia should use all other strategies available to them. This point of view is formulated for other communicatively impaired groups using AAC devices as well. For many users it is appropriate to use an AAC system as a backup to some other mode of communication (Murphy, Markova, Collins, & Moodie, 1996).

In addition to supporting "on-line communication", "off-line" communication also needs to be considered. For many people with aphasia it is important to prepare for a particular communicative situation, for instance for their doctor's appointment where they have to discuss complaints and medication, or for going to the hairdresser's and giving instructions for the preferred colour or style of haircut.

Not much is known about the interaction of natural speech with AAC strategies. On the one hand there is evidence to suggest that patients' natural language will improve after intensive training of communicative situations in which the use of AAC is prohibited (Pulvermuller et al., 2001), on the other hand, some researchers report improved verbal output associated with AAC training when using a device (Weinrich, 1995).

Vocabulary

For functional use, it is crucial that the vocabulary is relevant for the user's communicative needs. Often a vocabulary is a standard set (utterances, words, pictures, gestures etc.), thought to be a core set for communication (Bertoni, Stoffel, & Weniger, 1991; de Vries et al., 2001; Funnell & Allport, 1989; Stumpel et al., 1989; Verschaeve, 1998; Rao, 2001; Verschaeve & Wielaert, 1994). For many users, such a standard set does not meet the communicative need. Most vocabulary will never be used in functional settings, while it also lacks specific topics that are relevant for the individual. In those cases, the user will be reluctant to use the system.

For a personalised vocabulary it is necessary that it is continuously updated to reflect current needs. In this process of vocabulary selection, the therapist should work together with the client and their family and friends, interviewing them about communicative needs (Worrall, 1999). It is important to realise that partners who know the user very well, tend to "understand anyway". They sometimes do not see the need for certain kinds of vocabulary that may enhance communicative independence and enable the aphasic person to enter new communicative situations independently.

Information about the main topics in everyday communication is very important for building a relevant vocabulary for a client. Davidson et al. (2003) compared the everyday communication activities of healthy older people and older people with aphasia who were living in the community. Their observations revealed that many conversation topics were common in both groups, although people with aphasia tended to focus on the "here and now".

A vocabulary is often focused on information exchange, but other aspects of communication, e.g., "social talk", are important aspects as well. Users may need a vocabulary for topic introductions, items to prevent communication breakdown and to facilitate repair, strategies for story telling, greeting people, information about current situations, social closeness, and biographical information.

In the systems that are reported, several ways of accessing the vocabulary have been used: icons, pictures, written words, and combinations of these (Bertoni et al., 1991; de Vries et al., 2001; Funnell & Allport, 1989; Verschaeve, 1998; Weinrich, 1995).

The organisation of a vocabulary may be in topics, in a semantic hierarchy, alphabetically, or phonologically. There is no information about the selection of access systems for specific patients. It is largely unknown which systems are suitable for which patients.

Training

A person with aphasia, who is able to use a repertoire of AAC techniques in the clinician's room, often demonstrates limited use in daily life. One of the reasons for this might be a lack of appropriate training. There is a need for functional, pragmatic training, using role-play and simulations with a sufficient number of examples to promote generalisation and increase confidence. PACE therapy (Davis & Wilcox, 1981) provides a structured communicative situation in which the use of AAC can be optimised. However, communicative training inside the therapy room can still be experienced as very unnatural, and patients may need "in vivo training", using their skills in real-life communicative settings, coached by their aphasia therapist.

Fox, Moore Sohlberg, and Fried-Oken (2001) compared own-chosen communication topics with non-favourite topics in communication aid training in three aphasic patients. One of them benefited from choice of conversational topic in communication aid training, but this did not extend to natural environments.

An important issue is communicative flexibility: in using AAC strategies, the person with aphasia should be able to switch from one strategy to another, depending on the best way to convey a message. Yoshihata, Watamori, Chujo, and Masuyama (1998) investigated the ability to acquire mode interchange skills. Three participants with aphasia learned to use either a drawing or a gesture to ask for an object. None of the subjects spontaneously shifted from one mode to another, but they learned to do this on request.

Switching was trained using gestural prompts (rotation of the experimenter's thumb through 180 degrees). The ability to acquire this mode interchange skill varied considerably from person to person. These results point at the important role of the communication partners for facilitating nonverbal flexibility. Using alternate modes of communication largely depends on whether the communication partner provides the opportunity to employ acquired skills, or even actively stimulates the person with aphasia to do so. Therefore, the acceptance of alternative communication strategies on the part of familiar partners is essential.

The amount of time needed to learn a new system and to use this as an integral part of one's communicative behaviour should not be underestimated. A (non-aphasic) AAC user usually receives approximately 40 hours of therapy per year. This does not seem to be enough, compared to the 200 hours it is estimated to take to learn to speak English as a foreign language to the level of holding a basic conversation (Murphy et al., 1996). Evidently, training clients and their communication partners in functional settings is very time consuming.

Communication partners

In general, it has been observed that AAC users have difficulty initiating topics within interactions, and they tend to occupy a respondent's role. This seems to be true for many people with a severe aphasia, and it implies that the communication partner plays a central role: "Skilled communication partners can make the difference between successful and unsuccessful communication." (Garrett & Beukelman, 1992, p. 246). A skilled therapist displays behaviour that may enable an person with aphasia to communicate more effectively (Bryan, MacIntosh, & Brown, 1998) and includes:

- making specific requests for information;
- careful rephrasing of questions that are not understood;
- allowing enough time for the person to respond to a question;
- clarifying responses;
- guessing the meaning of the output;
- encouraging nonverbal communication.

This stresses the importance of the role of the communication partner, who will have to be trained to facilitate communicative strategies of his/her aphasic communication partner and to incorporate his/her new strategies into the communicative repertoire (Kagan, 1998).

For all AAC systems used, the communication partner should be a qualified "receiver". Systems that are not understood naturally by naive communicative partners, e.g., formal sign languages or pictorial systems, can only be used when communicating with people who have mastered the system.

Conclusions about low-tech aids

The factors described above as influencing the success of low-tech AAC in aphasia may be expected to play the same role when applied to high-tech communication devices. The most important lesson to be learned from the application of low-tech AAC seems to be the heterogeneity of the population, not only in the characteristics of aphasia, but also in cognitive abilities, communicative abilities and needs, motivation, and the communicative environment. This implies that AAC techniques should be individualised and "tailor-made", taking advantage of residual language skills and communicative strengths. The AAC tools should be adapted for use in personal communicative needs. Standard vocabularies are often too general and too restricted at the same time.

Clinicians will agree that they have far more tests and therapy materials to offer their clients disorder-oriented language therapy than to offer them AAC training. Therefore, their first option will often be a disorder-oriented approach. Also, quite understandably, many clinicians, clients, and spouses tend to reach for the highest possible goal of aphasia therapy: restoration of language comprehension and language production. As a result, AAC strategies are often seen as a "second", or maybe even "last" option, and they are mainly offered to people with a very severe aphasia, who might not be the best candidates for AAC intervention, because of restricted residual language processing and severe concomitant neuropsychological disorders.

At the same time, for patients with moderate or mild aphasia the use of AAC may not be considered, although they might be better candidates for AAC use, using AAC to support their spoken communication in daily life.

HIGH-TECH AAC INTERVENTION IN APHASIA

To our knowledge, there are no group studies investigating the use of communication aids by people with aphasia: hence little is known about the potential effect of electronic and computerised communication aids for aphasic communication. Most aids that are commercially available were developed for other groups: for children who do not develop spoken language, or for people with acquired dysarthria of varying aetiologies, e.g., stroke, ALS, Parkinson's disease, locked-in syndrome, multiple sclerosis, or traumatic brain injury. Occasionally these aids are used by people with aphasia.

High-tech communication aids designed for other client groups

An important characteristic of high-tech communication aids is that these machines can talk. Speech output may be either digitised or synthesised. Digitised speech is recorded with a microphone and stored digitally, therefore, it sounds natural. Synthesised speech is generated by software and sounds unnatural. When digitised speech is used, all speech output has to be pre-stored, and therefore it is less flexible. The advantage of synthesised speech is that new messages can be formulated and spoken. Individuals who are unable to formulate a message, but who can select whole messages, will typically use digitised speech, i.e., pre-stored messages.

The choice of the device often depends on the size of the vocabulary needed and the user's ability to retrieve stored messages. The Message Mate and the Dynamo (see Appendix) are devices that provide the option to store and retrieve messages in combination with speech output. The Message Mate, with a static display, is more restricted than the Dynamo, which has a dynamic display. In a dynamic display, more "levels" of messages can be included: a button may be used either to produce a message or to enter a new display, with a new set of messages. The person with aphasia who needs a large vocabulary will only benefit if he or she is able to navigate the system and to retrieve the target message relatively fast.

Communication aids may be text-based or icon-based. The Lightwriter (see Appendix) is a text-based communication aid with synthesised speech that is used occasionally by people with aphasia. The user should be able to formulate new messages and a high level of spelling is required. Therefore, the majority of people with aphasia will not be able to benefit from this device.

Iconic encoding enables the user to create messages by combining two and three icons. However, like formulating written messages, the use of iconic encoding will be difficult for the majority of clients with aphasia (Bertoni et al., 1991; Funnell & Allport, 1989). Beck and Fritz (1998) investigated whether persons with aphasia were able to learn iconic encoding. People with aphasia appeared to learn iconic encoding in a controlled recall task. Concrete messages were easier than abstract messages, both for aphasic and for non-aphasic participants. All persons with aphasia were able to learn the concrete messages; persons with good language comprehension were able to learn abstract messages at the one-icon level. There were no aphasic subjects who learned the abstract messages with two or three icons. Type of aphasia, level of abstraction, and length of icon sequence influenced learning. The authors concluded that it is probably better to offer dynamic displays (hierarchical vocabularies), since people with aphasia were much better at learning one-to-one relationships between icons and messages.

High-tech communication aids, specifically designed for aphasia

So far, many aphasiologists who have developed computerised systems to aid aphasic communication, have focused on developing prostheses for specific linguistic problems like word finding problems and problems in generating messages/sentences. In a sense, these "prosthetic systems" still are disorder-oriented, rather than communication-oriented, because they try to overcome a specific linguistic disorder. Recently, devices have been developed to support conversation. These have a functional orientation, aiming at the levels of activities and participation.

Devices aiding word finding.   The first computerised communication aid specifically designed for aphasia was described by Colby, Christinaz, Parkinson, Graham, and Karpf (1982). It requires restricted writing skills in combination with a simple system of word prediction. The system, running on a portable computer, was designed as a word finding prosthesis, a dynamic system using phonological and semantic information to identify a target word. When the user experiences difficulty finding a word, the display presents the following questions:

1. What is the topic area?
2. What is the first letter of the word?
3. What is the last letter of the word?
4. What letters are in the middle of the word?
5. What word does this word go with?

The user offers clues about the target word and the computer's reaction is a list of the "most probable words". This same concept of cueing and tapping the aphasic person's partial knowledge of a word that cannot be activated, is also used in a computerised therapy program for word finding, called "Multicue" (Doesborgh, van de Sandt-Koenderman, Dippel, van Harskamp, Koudstaal, & Visch-Brink, 2004 this issue; van Mourik & van de Sandt-Koenderman, 1992).

Another computer system for word finding was presented by Bruce and Howard (1987). In a naming task, the system provided the link between letters and sounds, for patients who were able to identify the first letter of a target word and who benefited from initial sound cueing. The patient found the initial letter, pressed it, and this was converted into a phoneme by the aid. Five patients for whom this conversion of letters into sounds was a missing link, were taught to use the system in five sessions. Four of them were significantly better in a naming task when they used the aid. The authors indicated that the system could be used in therapy, but when used as a prosthetic device, a smaller and portable version would be required.

Devices aiding sentence construction. C-VIC (Computerized Visual Communication; Steele, Weinrich, Wertz, Kleczewska, & Carlson, 1989) was designed specifically for aphasia, as an alternative communication system and as a therapeutic tool. Icons representing natural language lexical items (nouns, verbs, prepositions etc.) can be used to compose messages. C-VIC was developed over the years and in several studies a beneficial effect was reported (Steele et al., 1989; Shelton et al., 1996; Weinrich, 1995). Two patients with Broca's aphasia learned to produce SVO sentences with C-VIC syntax, and their verbal ability also improved considerably (Weinrich, 1995).

Shelton et al. (1996) found that in people with a global aphasia, there is a large variation in the ability to learn the system. While all patients did learn to use nouns, some people appeared unable to use verbs. This variability in verb processing in severe patients is also reported by other authors and probably depends on specific linguistic processes that may or may not be spared in severe aphasia (Koul & Harding, 1998).

The practical applications of C-VIC as an AAC system are restricted. Even people who are able to learn the system need extensive training over one or more years, resulting in a restricted vocabulary (e.g., 24 verbs, 150 nouns) with limited value for functional communication. People who had the system at home, used it for training purposes but never to communicate with family or friends.

The therapeutic efficacy of C-VIC is supported by two studies investigating the effectiveness of Lingraphica, the commercial version of C-VIC, which is described as an extensive toolbox of specially designed, interactive multimodal materials for use with and by people with aphasia (Aftonomos et al., 1997). Lingraphica was used with 23 clients and most participants showed improvement in multiple modalities, including verbal. In a second study (Aftonomos, Appelbaum, & Steele, 1999), 60 chronic participants were treated with Linguagraphica. The therapist chose the exercises following an algorithm. The focus was on functional improvement outside the clinic. In addition to the therapy sessions, participants used the system at home, exploring its possibilities for typically 2 hours per day. A large majority of participants showed significant improvements in both language impairment and communicative function, regardless of time post onset.

Both C-VIC and Lingraphica run on a PC. No small, portable devices are described.

Linebarger, Schwartz, Romania, Kohn, and Stephens (2000) describe a communication system, CS, running on a PC as a processing prosthesis for people with agrammatism. While C-VIC provides word finding assistance (using icons) during sentence construction, this system concentrates on producing longer utterances without aiding word finding. It was conceived as a tool to overcome processing limitations, rather than to replace grammatical encoding. The user speaks into a microphone, and a coloured shape represents the recorded chunk, which can be touched to play the utterance back. By moving these shapes into an assembly area at the top of the screen, the chunks can be combined into larger structures: sentences and texts. The system significantly facilitated syntactic structure for five of the six participants. In a subsequent study, CS was used for communication using the Internet (Linebarger, Schwartz, Kantner, & McCall, 2002)

Devices aiding conversation.   Talksbac, a system running on a Macintosh Powerbook with a built-in speech synthesiser (Waller, Brodie, & Cairns, 1998), can be described as a conversation aid. An adaptive knowledge base assists in conversation by predicting the communication partner, the topic of conversation, and probable sentences and story titles. The information (messages and stories) is personalised by the therapist. The authors report that partners were unable to anticipate the conversational needs of the client with aphasia.

Four persons with Broca's aphasia, who were at least 1 year post onset, were included in the study. An analysis of videotaped conversations between the participants and familiar and unfamiliar partners showed that three of them benefited from using Talksbac. For one of the clients the system was too slow. The participants showed an increase in topic initiations and expansions, together with a decrease in responses and fewer communication breakdowns when using Talksbac.

PCAD, a Personal Communication Assistant for Dysphasic People, was specifically designed for aphasia by an international team of software specialists, aphasia specialists, and AAC specialists. The team decided to build a flexible aid that could be easily adapted to the user's personal needs and that was small enough to be really portable. As a hardware platform, a commercially available palmtop computer was chosen (Hewlett Packard 620 LX), with a colour touch screen and sound output. Based on the view that people with a severe aphasia constitute a very heterogeneous population, the aid was devised as a modular system. This was felt to be necessary because people with different types of aphasia and varying levels of linguistic processing, with different levels of cognitive functioning and a range of communicative skills and communicative needs, were expected to need different systems. The software, called Touchspeak provides the following modules:

- A hierarchically organised vocabulary; the therapist may include photos, pictures, symbols, words, and sentences. Here, a personal vocabulary is built with personalised or standard messages. The user addresses the items by clicking the computer screen, thus navigating the hierarchical system, and activating a message. These messages can be "spoken" out by the computer.
- Speech output, using either digitised speech, or synthesised speech.
- A typing option, where the user can type (parts of) words/utterances. The message can be stored in a "gallery" to use on later occasions.
- A drawing option, for those clients who use communicative drawings. The user can draw (or write) directly on the colour screen. As in the typing option, drawings can be stored in the gallery and used again in new communicative situations.
- The news page is a page where recent information can be typed in. Text and/or pictures are stored in categories. This option may be used by relatives to type information that the aphasic user can refer to, when communicating with others.
- A message bar, at the bottom of the screen, is where one or more messages from the hierarchical vocabulary can be stored temporarily during conversation. The message bar is also a tool that can be used for off-line communication.
- The phonemic cueing option: only the first sound(s) of a word or utterance is sounded out; this option is useful for those who prefer to say the message themselves, if possible.

The system has to be configured for each client. The clinician, the client, and his/her family decide together which modules are relevant. These are installed on the palmtop. The therapist and the user decide on the communicative goals, and together they build a relevant vocabulary.

In a multiple-case study, 22 people with aphasia in three European countries, received PCAD training; they all learned to operate the aid, and 17 of them used the device functionally, in everyday life, for pre-set communicative goals, such as shopping or telephone conversations with family, or with unfamiliar people like the hairdresser or the taxi-company (van de Sandt-Koenderman et al., submitted). All clients used the hierarchical vocabulary with a personalised set of messages, related to their personal communicative goals. The other options were not used by all clients: The clients used the same device for varying communicative goals (Wiegers, van de Sandt-Koenderman, & Wielaert, 2002).

Not all clients chose to use speech output. One client, for instance, used the system more or less "off-line", preparing for communicative situations by typing specific messages. She used these messages in functional communication by reading them aloud, because she preferred to use her own voice. Another client, who was unable to speak spontaneously, used the microphone to record short messages. For instance she recorded the utterance "hello this is XX speaking", to use when answering the phone. Although the effect on her communicative efficiency may seem small, the emotional effect of being able to answer the phone with her own voice was valued by the client.

Nine months after the intervention, the six Dutch clients who learned to use PCAD in functional settings were interviewed. Four of them reported that they still used the aid in communicative settings. For one client, a longer follow-up was available. He used PCAD in functional settings as long as 2 years after the intervention (Wiegers et al., 2002). Since 2001, the device has been commercially available in the UK and in the Netherlands under the name Touchspeak (see Appendix).

Conclusions about high-tech aids

The use of high-tech communication aids in aphasia rehabilitation is restricted and with the exception of the C-VIC research group, no aphasiologists have been developing and refining a high-tech AAC system, reporting their results in the literature. The therapeutic value of C-VIC has been established for all types of aphasia, regardless of time post onset. However, as a communication device, it has limitations because aiding sentence construction, as in C-VIC, has limited value for on-line use in communicative situations. The process of formulating messages is time-consuming, while the communicative value of correct syntax is not very high. For off-line processing the situation may be different, but there are no studies reporting on the effect of C-VIC on off-line communication.

Aiding word finding seems much more powerful, especially for people who have some information about the word form. However, in this area there are only two relatively old studies with non-portable machines.

Systems that are oriented to communication in everyday life, like PCAD/Touchspeak and Talksbac, provide ready-made utterances that can be used in conversations. Talksbac uses written language as the modality to address the vocabulary. In PCAD/Touchspeak more options are available: written words, photos, drawings, pictographs. The organisation of these messages is hierarchical. In the PCAD project the client could decide which messages he or she needed, and where the message should be represented in the hierarchy.

Another way of organising a vocabulary was developed for other groups, but this has not been tested with aphasic users. Scriptalker, for instance (Dye, Alm, Arnott, Harper, & Morrison, 1998) uses a graphic, situational organisation of the messages, which might be beneficial for certain groups of aphasic people. The user may click parts of a situation depicted on the screen, thus entering specific conversational scripts and its messages. For instance, when clicking on the table in a restaurant scene, the script for communicating with the waiter becomes available, with messages like: choosing from the menu, asking for the bill, etc.

The modularity of PCAD/Touchspeak reflects the heterogeneity of the aphasic population. The modules are based on the low-tech AAC options that have been used so far: writing, drawing, and book systems with pictures, symbols, or written words. Gesturing was—for obvious reasons—not included.

Good writing skills are crucial, because these enable a client to produce new messages. However the PCAD project shows that even a restricted vocabulary of ready-made utterances for a specific situation can be of use. A vocabulary for buying clothes, for instance, seems to be very restricted, but its role for the individual user may be very important, because it enables him/her to go shopping independently. As a result, the communicative device may enhance participation for this specific situation, but it may also reduce anxiety in other situations and serve as a tool to stimulate the person with aphasia to participate independently, initiating communication more often (Wiegers et al., 2002).

DISCUSSION

This review of the state of the art in the field of AAC and aphasia points at two main factors that may explain why the development and implementation of computerised communication aids for aphasia has been relatively slow.

First, the work of clinicians who use high-tech or low-tech AAC applications has rarely been published in the literature on clinical management of aphasia. Detailed case studies are scarce, and efficacy studies are virtually non-existent. Consequently, many therapists have a limited view of AAC, and those who try to develop a structured approach cannot use published material and seem to have to re-invent the wheel over and over again. This makes it very difficult to specify the system requirements for communication aids for aphasia.

Second, developing a communication aid is an enormous task, for which limited resources are available. Because of the heterogeneity of the population, all solutions will only be useful for a subpart of the aphasic group, so the investment of time and money is huge, for a small group of users. Compared to developing a word processing programme for healthy people, the development of an aid for a subgroup of the aphasic population is extremely expensive. In the meantime, the technological developments will go on, and any device risks being outdated before its development is complete.

However, there is a moral obligation for aphasia therapists to explore the benefits of new technologies and to use them to improve the client's quality of life, by enhancing participation. What needs to be done if we want to use the potential of computer technology adequately to build AAC devices for people with aphasia?

First of all, therapists will have to widen their horizons, and develop a new view of AAC strategies in general, and their role in aphasia rehabilitation in particular. AAC should not be seen as a last resort for clients who do not benefit from disorder-oriented therapy. It should be an integral part of aphasia rehabilitation for all people with aphasia.

Second, the application of AAC interventions should be investigated and reported in the literature. Improving language functioning to achieve a higher level of verbal communication in everyday life is an important goal in aphasia therapy. Most communication partners of the person with aphasia are healthy speakers and, therefore, improvement of natural language processes has a high priority in aphasia rehabilitation. However, we also know that chronic aphasia is a lifetime condition, even if considerable linguistic progress can be achieved. Therefore, the individual has to adapt to his or her new situation and any helpful strategy should be used to improve communicative skills. To define these helpful strategies, it is important to focus on the levels of activity and participation rather than on the impairment level (WHO, 2001) not only for severe patients, but also for persons with a moderate or mild aphasia.

Furthermore, we will have to accept that it is impossible to build communication systems with a vocabulary that can replace natural language for all communicative roles. Any system that tries to do this will fail. A normal speaker has a vocabulary of at least 50,000 words, but he or she may know as many as 250,000 words (Aitchison, 1987). Most of these words, can be retrieved in a fraction of a second; furthermore, the normal speaker can combine them into meaningful utterances without effort, and produce these utterances at a speed of 2–3 words per second (Levelt, 1989). Like any aid, a communication aid can never compete with the unimpaired function, in this case with natural language. It is a second-best solution, and it will not be used functionally, unless the user gains more than he or she has to invest.

A better orientation would be to accept that no AAC strategy or AAC device will ever be as efficient as natural language. The user has to decide whether a specific device meets his or her needs to such an extent, that he or she wants to take the trouble to use it.

A communication aid should be personally tailored, both in what it can do and in the vocabulary included. The PCAD/Touchspeak project offers an example of this approach. It aimed at developing a highly flexible communication aid and therefore a modular system was developed, with a personalised vocabulary. The approach implies that the clients are interviewed about their personal communicative needs, and that the therapist and the client make shared decisions regarding the role and the specifications of the AAC applications (Worrall, 1999; Worrall & Frattali, 2000). They may come up with imaginative solutions for specific communicative goals and become more aware of what technology might have to offer, now and in the future. These solutions should be reported in the literature enabling AAC research—both high-tech and low-tech—in order to further develop the field of AAC and aphasia.

Research into AAC and aphasia in general is needed in order to build and refine computerised communication aids for individuals with aphasia, although questions about whether high-tech solutions are more beneficial than low-tech solutions will not be addressed easily, because we do not know how beneficial low-tech strategies are for aphasic communication.

Research questions expected to be important are:

- Selection of patients: which patients may benefit from which systems, and can we specify the characteristics of ''good candidates'' for specific devices/strategies? Can we identify cognitive and linguistic skills that are prerequisites for adequate use?
- Stage of recovery: at what time do we introduce AAC? Is it possible to benefit from AAC in the acute phase, or do we have to wait until 6 or 12 months post onset, before introducing a device/strategies?

- What is the relation between use of AAC and recovery of language functions? Does disorder-oriented therapy need to precede AAC intervention?
- What is the advantage of high-tech solutions over low-tech AAC strategies?

After reviewing the state of the art in computerised communication aids for persons with aphasia, it has become clear that every aid will be used in combination with other low-tech AAC strategies and, of course (if possible) with speaking. Using a computer system in addition to other ways of communicating may have several advantages:

- A computer system is dynamic and may be easily adapted to personal needs.
- A vocabulary needs to be adapted regularly, because the communicative needs of a person with aphasia change over time. Adding or deleting messages, or changing the organisation, can be done easily in a computerised system, and the system will still look "new"; in contrast, a well-organised communication book or a notepad will become disordered and grimy/shabby over time.
- If needed, a computer can produce speech output, sometimes even the person with aphasia's own production can be recorded (e.g., using reading aloud) to be used in communicative settings.
- The computer is a powerful tool for off-line communication: the user may build the messages he or she expects to need in a certain communicative situation, and spend as much time as needed, till he/she is satisfied with the result. These messages may be stored, and used later in functional settings. Typing on a computer is often more satisfactory, because self-corrections are made easily and do not leave traces, unlike writing.
- The user's motivation may grow when high-tech solutions are used. Many users of book systems are reluctant to use them in communicative settings, while most clients in the PCAD study were enthusiastic about the device: they felt that an of-the-shelf palmtop computer is not associated with a disability. Many of them did not hesitate to use it in unfamiliar settings, and this effect may be used as a powerful tool to reach communicative independence. A sophisticated device may also help the individual to feel more secure in addressing unfamiliar communication partners, whose reaction will be more positive. Therefore the device may very well have a catalytic effect on the communication partner as well.

These possible advantages may serve to encourage clinicians to move forward. The effort to develop computerised communication aids seems worthwhile, provided that the device is tested in communicative settings, and that the results are carefully documented and reported. Clinicians should also stay alert to see what happens in the field of high-tech AAC for other client groups. Specific communicative needs of persons with aphasia may sometimes be met by devices for other groups and these devices should be tested by people with aphasia. An example is a new device for people with dyslexia for instance, the ReadingPen (see Appendix). This is a pen that, when moved over written text, will read this text aloud. This system might prove to be a powerful tool for persons with a Broca's aphasia and deep dyslexia, associated with a relatively good auditory comprehension of sentences. Using the ReadingPen might, for instance, enable them to read their mail independently.

In conclusion, the use of high-tech computerised communication aids by people with aphasia is a promising new route to explore. Aphasiologists have only just begun to see the possibilities offered by technology. It is important to develop and test new systems and, last but not least, report the efficacy of functional use in the literature, so that these devices can find their way into the daily practice of aphasia rehabilitation.

REFERENCES

Aftonomos, L. B., Appelbaum, J. S., & Steele, R. D. (1999). Improving outcomes for persons with aphasia in advanced community-based treatment programs. *Stroke, 30*, 1370–1379.

Aftonomos, L. B., Steele, R. D., & Wertz, R. T. (1997). Promoting recovery in chronic aphasia with an interactive technology. *Archives of Physical Medicine, 78*, 841–846.

Aitchison, J. (1987). *Words in the mind.* Oxford: Basil Blackwell Ltd.

Beck, A. R., & Fritz, H. (1998). Can people with aphasia learn iconic codes? *Augmentative and Alternative Communication, 14*, 184–195.

Bertoni, B., Stoffel, A. M., & Weniger, D. (1991). Communicating with pictographs: A graphic approach to the improvement of communicative interactions. *Aphasiology, 5*, 341–353.

Bruce, C., & Howard, D. (1987). Computer-generated phonemic cues: An effective aid for naming in aphasia. *British Journal of Disorders of Communication, 22*, 191–201.

Bryan, K., MacIntosh, J., & Brown, D. (1998). Extending conversation analysis to non-verbal communication. *Aphasiology, 12*, 179–188.

Cicerone, K. D., Dahlberg, C., Kalmar, K., Langenbahn, D. M., Malec, J. F., Bergquist, T. F., et al. (2000). Evidence-based cognitive rehabilitation: Recommendations for clinical practice. *Archives of Physical Medicine and Rehabilitation, 81*, 1596–1615.

Colby, K. M., Christinaz D., Parkinson, R. C., Graham, S., & Karpf, C. (1982). A word-finding computer program with a dynamic lexical-semantic memory for patients with anomia using an intelligent speech prosthesis. *Brain and Language, 14*, 272–281.

Cruice, M., Worrall, L., Hickson, L., & Murison, R. (2003). Finding a focus for quality of life with aphasia: Social and emotional health, and psychological well-being. *Aphasiology, 17*, 333–353.

Davidson, B., Worrall, L., & Hickson, L. (2003). Identifying the communication activities of older people with aphasia: Evidence from naturalistic observation. *Aphasiology, 17*, 243–264.

Davis, G. A., & Wilcox, M. J. (1981). Incorporating parameters of natural conversation in aphasia treatment. In R. Chapey (Ed.), *Language intervention strategies in adult aphasia* (pp. 169–195). Baltimore: Williams & Wilkins.

de Vries, L. A., Stumpel, H., Stoutjesdijk O., & Barf, H. (2001). *Het Taalzakboek.* Lisse: Swets & Zeitlinger BV.

Doesborgh, S. J. C., van de Sandt-Koenderman, W. M. E., Dippel, D. W. J., van Harskamp, F., Koudstaal, P. J., & Visch-Brink, E. G. (2004). Cues on request. The efficacy of Multicue, a computer program for word finding therapy. *Aphasiology, 18*(3), 213–222.

Dye, R., Alm, N., Arnott, J. L., Harper, G., & Morrison, A. I. (1998). A script-based AAC system for transactional interaction. *Natural Language Engineering, 4*, 57–71.

Feyereisen, P., Barter, D., Goossens, M., & Clerebaut, N. (1988). Gestures and speech in referential communication by aphasic subjects: Channel use and efficiency. *Aphasiology, 2*, 21–32.

Fox, L. E., Moore Sohlberg, M., & Fried-Oken, M. (2001). Effects of conversational topic choice on outcomes of augmentative communication intervention for adults with aphasia. *Aphasiology, 15*, 171–200.

Funnell, E., & Allport, A. (1989). Symbolically speaking: Communicating with Bliss symbols in aphasia. *Aphasiology, 3*, 279–300.

Garrett, K. L., & Beukelman, D. R. (1992). Augmentative communication approaches for persons with severe aphasia. In K. Yorkston (Ed.), *Augmentative communication in the medical setting* (pp. 245–321). Tucson, AZ: Communication Skill Builders.

Garrett, K. L., & Huth, C. (2002). The impact of graphic contextual information and instruction on the conversational behaviours of a person with severe aphasia. *Aphasiology, 16*, 523–536.

Hier, D. B., & Mohr, J. P. (1977). Incongruous oral and written naming. *Brain and Language, 4*, 208–235.

Hux, K. D., Beukelman, R., & Garrett, K. L. (1994). Augmentative and alternative communication for persons with aphasia. In R. Chapey (Ed.), *Language intervention strategies in adult aphasia, Third edition* (pp. 338–357. Baltimore: Williams & Wilkins.

Hux, K. D., Manasse, N., Weiss, A., & Beukelman, D. R. (2001). Augmentative and alternative communication for persons with aphasia. In R. Chapey (Ed.), *Language intervention strategies in aphasia and related neurogenic communication disorders, Fourth edition* (pp. 675–687). Baltimore/Philadelphia: Lippincott Williams & Wilkins.

Kagan, A. (1998). Supported conversation for adults with aphasia: Methods and resources for training conversation partners. *Aphasiology*, *12*, 816–830.

Katz, R. C. (2001). Computer applications in aphasia treatment. In R. Chapey (Ed.), *Language intervention strategies in aphasia and related neurogenic communication disorders, Fourth edition* (pp. 718–741). Baltimore/Philadelphia: Lippincott Williams & Wilkins.

Katz, R. C., & Wertz, R. T. (1997). The efficacy of computer-provided reading treatment for chronic aphasic adults. *Journal of Speech, Language and Hearing Research*, *40*, 493–507.

Koul, R. K., & Harding, R. (1998). Identification and production of graphic symbols by individuals with aphasia: Efficacy of a software application. *Augmentative and Alternative Communication*, *14*, 11–23.

Kraat, A. W. (1990). Augmentative and alternative communication: Does it have a future in aphasia rehabilitation? *Aphasiology*, *4*, 321–338.

Levelt, W. J. M. (1989). *Speaking: From intention to articulation*. Cambridge, MA: MIT Press.

Light, J., & Lindsay, P. (1991). Cognitive science and augmentative and alternative communication. *Augmentative and Alternative Communication*, *1*, 186–203.

Linebarger, M. C., Schwartz, M. F., Kantner, T. R., & McCall, D. (2002). Promoting access to the Internet in aphasia. *Brain and Language*, *83*, 169–172.

Linebarger, M. C., Schwartz, M. F., Romania, J. R., Kohn, S. E., & Stephens, D. L. (2000). Grammatical encoding in aphasia: Evidence from a processing prosthesis. *Brain and Language*, *75*, 416–427.

Lyon, J. (1995). Drawing: Its value as a communication aid for adults with aphasia. *Aphasiology*, *9*, 33–95.

Murphy, J., Markova, I., Collins, S., & Moodie, E. (1996). AAC systems: obstacles to effective use. *European Journal of Disorders of Communication*, *31*, 31–44.

Pedersen, P. M., Vinter, K., & Olsen, T. S. (2001). Improvement of oral naming by unsupervised computerised rehabilitation. *Aphasiology*, *15*, 151–169.

Pulvermuller, F., Neininger, B., Elbert, T., Mohr, B., Rockstroh, B., Koebbel, P. et al. (2001). Constraint-induced therapy of chronic aphasia after stroke. *Stroke*, *32*, 1621–1626.

Rao, P. R. (2001). Use of Amer Ind Code by persons with severe aphasia. In R. Chapey (Ed.), *Language intervention strategies in aphasia and related neurogenic communication disorders, Fourth edition* (pp. 688–702). Baltimore/Philadelphia: Lippincott Williams & Wilkins.

Robey, R. R. (1994). The efficacy of treatment for aphasic persons: A meta-analysis. *Brain and Language*, *47*, 585–608.

Robey, R. R., & Schultz, M. (1998). A model for conducting clinical-outcome research: An adaptation of the standard protocol for use in aphasiology. *Aphasiology*, *12*, 787–810.

Scott, C., & Byng, S. (1989). Computer assisted remediation of a homophone comprehension disorder in surface dyslexia. *Aphasiology*, *3*, 301–320.

Semenza, S., Cippolotti, L., & Denes, G. (1992). Reading aloud in jargonaphasia: An unusual dissociation in speech output. *Journal of Neurology, Neurosurgery and Psychiatry*, *55*, 205–208.

Shelton, J. R., Weinrich, M., McCall, D., & Cox, D. M. (1996). Differentiating globally aphasic patients: Data from in-depth language assessments and production training using C-VIC. *Aphasiology*, *10*, 319–342.

Stachowiak, F. J. (1993). Computer-based aphasia therapy with the Lingware/STACH system. In F. J. Stachowiak, G. Deloche, R. Kaschel, H. Kremin, P. North, L. Pizzamiglio et al. (Eds.), *Developments in the assessment and rehabilitation of brain-damaged patients* (pp. 354–380). Tubingen: Gunter Narr Verlag.

Steele, R. D., Weinrich, M., Wertz, R.T., Kleczewska, M., & Carlson, G. (1989). Computer based visual communication as an alternative communication system and therapeutic tool. *Neuropsychologia*, *27*, 409–426.

Stumpel, M. J. E. J., van Dijk, H., Messing-Peterson, J. J. M., & de Vries, L. A. (1989). Systeem voor training van afasiepatienten. In E. G. Visch-Brink, F. van Harskamp, & D. de Boer (Eds.), *Afasietherapie* (pp. 182–192). Amsterdam: Swets & Zeitlinger.

van de Sandt-Koenderman, W. M. E., & Visch-Brink, E. G. (1993). Experiences with Multicue. In F. J. Stachowiak, G. Deloche, R. Kaschel, H. Kremin, P. North, L. Pizzamiglio et al. (Eds.), *Developments in the assessment and rehabilitation of brain-damaged patients* (pp. 347–351). Tubingen: Gunter Narr Verlag.

van Mourik, M., & van de Sandt-Koenderman, W. M. E. (1992). Multicue. *Aphasiology*, *6*, 179–183.

van Mourik, M.., Verschaeve, M., Boon, P., Paquier, P., & van Harskamp, F. (1992). Cognition in global aphasia: Indicators for therapy. *Aphasiology*, *5*, 491–499.

Verschaeve, M. A. W. (1998). Het Gespreksboek als ondersteunend communicatiemiddel. *Logopedie en Foniatrie*, *11*, 81–85.

Verschaeve, M. A. H. & Wielaert S. M. (1994). Ondersteunde communicatie bij afasie. *Logopedie en Foniatrie*, *5*, 151–153.

Visch-Brink, E. G. (1999). *Words in action*. Rotterdam: Erasmus University Rotterdam.

Visch-Brink, E. G., van Harskamp, F., van Amerongen, N. M., Wielaert, S. M., & van de Sandt-Koenderman, W. M. E. (1993). A multidisciplinary approach to aphasia therapy. In A. L. Holland & M. M. Forbes (Eds.), *Aphasia Treatment, world perspectives*. San Diego, CA: Singular Publishing Group, Inc.

Waller, A., Brodie, J., & Cairns, A. Y. (1998). Evaluating Talksbac, a predictive communication device for nonfluent adults with aphasia. *International Journal of Language and Communication Disorders*, *33*, 45–70.

Weinrich, M. (1995). Training on an iconic communication system for severe aphasia can improve natural language production. *Aphasiology*, *9*, 343–364.

WHO (2001). *ICF, International classification of functioning, disability and health*. Geneva: WHO.

Whurr, R., Lorch, M., & Nye, C. A. (1992). Meta-analysis of studies carried out between 1946 and 1988 concerned with the efficacy of speech and language therapy treatment for aphasic patients. *European Journal of Disorders of Communication*, *27*, 1–18.

Wiegers, J. J., van de Sandt-Koenderman, W. M. E., & Wielaert, S. M. (2002). "Ik heb afasie, ik kan niet praten. Ik gebruik nu een computer om mee te praten." PCAD, een elektronisch hulpmiddel voor mensen met afasie. *Logopedie en Foniatrie*, *74*, 180–185.

Worrall, L. (1999). *Functional Communication Therapy Planner (FCTP)*. Oxon, UK: Winslow Press Ltd.

Worrall, L. E., & Frattali, C. M. (Eds.). (2000). *Neurogenic communication disorders: A functional approach*. New York: Thieme.

Yoshihata, H., Watamori, T., Chujo, T., & Masuyama, K. (1998). Acquisition and generalization of mode interchange skills in people with severe aphasia. *Aphasiology*, *12*, 1035–1046.

APPENDIX

Communication aids

Lightwriter: www.toby-churchill.com
Message Mate: www.words-plus.com
Dynamo: www.dynavoxsys.com & www.sunrisemedical.com
ReadingPen: www.wizcomtech.com

PCAD/Touchspeak (UK):
Richard Hill & Associates, 33 Shamrock Way, Southgate, London, N14 5SA, UK.
Tel +44 208 368 6219
Email: gjb30@dial.pipex.com
Website: www.ace-centre.org.uk/html/research/pcad/pcadproj.html

PCAD/Touchspeak (The Netherlands, Germany):
RdgKompagne, Winthontlaan 200, 3526 KV Utrecht, The Netherlands.
Tel +31 30 2870564
Email: info@rdgkompagne.nl
Website: www.rdgkompagne.nl

APHASIOLOGY, 2004, *18* (3), 265–280

Accessible Internet training package helps people with aphasia cross the digital divide

Jennifer Egan, Linda Worrall, and Dorothea Oxenham

The University of Queensland, Brisbane, Australia

Background: The Internet is a source of information, communication, and leisure opportunities for people with aphasia. However, accessible training is one of several barriers for people with aphasia in using the Internet.
Aims: This study developed and trialled special aphasia-friendly Internet training materials for people with aphasia.
Methods & Procedures: A total of 20 people with aphasia were matched with volunteer tutors. The tutor–student pairs met for six lessons. Pre- and post-test Internet skills assessments were conducted and attitudinal questionnaires were completed. The training materials were based on Microsoft Internet Explorer 5.5 and consisted of a tutor's manual and a manual for the Internet student with aphasia. These materials are available as a free download from: http://www.shrs.uq.edu.au/cdaru/aphasiagroups/
Outcomes & Results: Significant differences between pre and post scores were found and participants reached a range of levels of independence following the training. The majority reported favourable outcomes.
Conclusions. Results indicated that it was possible for people with aphasia to learn to use the Internet when they were taught in a one-to-one teaching situation with the use of accessible training manuals.

The term "digital divide" is increasingly used to describe the social implications of unequal access by some sectors of the community to information and communications technology and to the acquisition of necessary skills (*A strategic framework ##*, 2001). People with disabilities are one of these groups. The Internet has the potential for reducing barriers to information and communication and employment opportunities, and is particularly relevant to people with disabilities and others who have been "under-represented or underserved by traditional information, communication and educational systems" (Stoddard & Nelson, 2001, p.7). Tim Berners-Lee, who is attributed with being the inventor of the Internet, asserts that the power of the web is in its universality and that access by everyone regardless of a disability is an essential aspect (*The World Wide Web Consortium [W3C]*, 2001). However, Owens, Lamb, and Keller (2001) highlighted concerns about the actual usage of information technology by people with disabilities. Indeed, a 1998 population survey in America found that Americans with disabilities are less than half as likely as their counterparts to own a computer, and they are about one-quarter as likely to use the Internet (Kaye, 2000).

Address correspondence to: A/Prof Linda Worrall, Communication Disability in Ageing Research Unit, Department of Speech Pathology and Audiology, The University of Queensland, Brisbane, QLD 4072, Australia. Email l.worrall@uq.edu.au

     DOI:10.1080/02687030344000562

The increasing reliance on the Internet for information delivery and access has made it necessary for governments to develop strategies that ensure equal communications access for people with disabilities. The Australian Government's Online Strategy provides a basis for improving public access to a wide range of government services, especially by people who live in regional, rural, and remote areas, or older Australians and people with disabilities (*A strategic framework ##*, 2001). Furthermore, a number of other initiatives, including those of the Office of Government Online, the National Office of Information Economy, and the Human Rights and Equal Opportunity Commission are committed to making information, particularly electronic information, accessible to people with disabilities (*Commonwealth Disability Strategy*, 2001). These initiatives indicate a recognition that web developers need to comply with universal web design standards (*W3C*, 2001). Disability groups that have a history of self-advocacy have been effective in challenging inequities in the area of website accessibility. For example Maguire vs SOCOG (2000) created a legal precedent, in the case of a blind person who was successful in bringing a complaint concerning web inaccessibility against the Sydney Organising Committee for the Olympic Games, and in doing so, established that the Australian Disability Act covers website design (*Website found to be discriminatory*, 2000) In the case of people with aphasia, website accessibility has been recently addressed by Egan and Worrall (2001) who have produced Web Development Guidelines for people with aphasia.

The development of accessibility initiatives in the area of website design is an essential step in bridging the digital divide for people with aphasia. Realistically this must be regarded as a long-term endeavour that will involve policing of the web by people with aphasia and their advocates. It must also be stated that professionals who advocate fully accessible websites, without considering training and support needs, may be dangling a pot of gold without providing instructions as to how to get it! It is a concern that to date there has been little research on the training needs of people with disabilities, considering that a major barrier to computer and Internet access for people with disabilities is lack of training and support (Owens et al., 2001).

With regard to people with aphasia, Elman (2001) has flagged the importance of addressing digital divide barriers by stating that barriers to the Internet must be overcome for people with aphasia to achieve full participation in the digital economy. Effective training is therefore essential in order for people with aphasia to achieve the benefits of online communication.

BARRIERS TO INTERNET TRAINING FOR PEOPLE WITH APHASIA

Aphasia is primarily a communication disability that is characterised by degrees of impairment to the four modalities of verbal expression, auditory comprehension, and reading and writing abilities. A person with aphasia may be disadvantaged by these impairments in a training situation, because they may be unable to comprehend verbal instructions, understand written instructions, ask questions, or write homework notes. Other barriers to Internet training may be caused by stroke-induced symptoms, which may accompany aphasia, such as psychosocial changes, cognitive impairments, and sensori-motor impairments such as paralysis and apraxia. Psychosocial changes such as an altered self-image and feelings of confusion, misery, anger, loss, and intense frustration (Jordan & Kaiser, 1996) may create social access barriers for people with aphasia who may wish to attend public or private Internet training classes. Cognitive impairments such as a difficulty with sequencing steps to complete an activity, short-term memory loss, limited problem-solving capacity, and an altered capacity to monitor social behaviour (Peng, Adams, & Gentile, 1998) may also create barriers to training opportunities. Although people with aphasia do not usually require extensive assistive technology to use computers, it is possible that apraxia or muscle weakness may cause difficulty when using a standardised mouse and keyboard.

Age-related declines in cognition must also be addressed as an additional barrier for people with aphasia, many of whom are in the age categories of young-old (age 60–74 years) and old-old (age 75–89 years) (Echt, Morrell, & Park, 1998). A study by Morrell and Echt reports that older adults require more time than younger adults to acquire computer skills, usually commit more errors when performing computer tasks, and require more assistance than younger adults (Morrell & Echt, 1996). Morrell and Echt also suggested that age-related declines in cognitive abilities such as perceptual speed, verbal and spatial working memory, and text comprehension, play significant roles in age-related differences in computer skill acquisition (Echt et al., 1998). The ability to operate hardware may also be compromised as with advanced age and disability, mouse use becomes increasingly inaccurate (Riviere & Thakor, 1996).

Pillay (2000) refers to Internet students of older generations as "technological migrants", in that they are venturing into a world where many things are unfamiliar and another younger group holds a position of expertise and power. Older people with aphasia, then, are technological migrants with a complex communication disability.

An overview of existing Internet training opportunities reveals that most computer training materials have been designed for younger learners and that text is the most common presentation format for computer instructions (Echt et al., 1998). In fact, it appears probable that mainstream Internet training opportunities remain inaccessible to people with aphasia for the following reasons:

- Many bookshops are stocked with a variety of Internet training texts for beginners. These texts are designed for self-directed learning. They are designed using text instructions, computer terminology and supported with graphics of the Internet screen. Such texts are generally inaccessible to people with aphasia, due to literacy disability, and general inexperience with computers.
- Internet classes at public venues such as libraries usually cater for groups of all ages and there is an expectation that people keep pace with the class. The barriers for people with aphasia in this situation include literacy disability, auditory comprehension difficulties, and the time needed to ask for clarification, repetition, and individual help. The pressure to fit in with non-disabled people in an environment that demands a "real time" learning response is likely to be intimidating and may result in feelings of failure for people with aphasia.
- Private tuition as an option for Internet training raises the issue of economic barriers for people with aphasia.
- Online tutorials and CD rom tutorials are popular, however they cater for those people who already have some proficiency with a computer. Many people with aphasia have no experience with computer software or hardware. The barriers encountered with this training option are inexperience with computers and the lack of exposure to the specialised lexicon of technology terms used in such tutorials.

CONSIDERATIONS IN INTERNET TRAINING METHODS AND INSTRUCTIONAL DESIGN FOR PEOPLE WITH APHASIA

A recent literature review of computer and Internet training for people with disabilities conceded that there are some gaps in the documentation of the design and delivery of Internet training for computer users with disabilities and those who support them (Owens et al., 2001). As deficits in perceptual speed, working memory, and text comprehension are also experienced in older people, albeit to a lesser degree, this research drew on literature related to instructional design and training methods for older people. In a study of older adults using word-processing tasks, it was found that lack of time pressure resulted in superior performance, regardless of age (Charness, Schumann, & Boritz, cited in Echt et al., 1998). It is therefore advisable that people with aphasia be allowed to learn at their own pace in a training situation. For many reasons previously cited, it is probable that online learning or group learning in a classroom situation will be too challenging for most people with aphasia. If a self-directed learning model using text-based materials also proves too difficult, it would seem practical to use a face-to-face hands-on instruction method. Using this method, the participant observes as procedures are demonstrated. During the demonstration, the tutor and participant progress systematically through tasks, the tutor highlights key points, and after the demonstration, the tutor can prompt the participant to complete the task (Clothier, 1996). This self-paced one-to-one method is especially suitable to learning the Internet, as a participant may be confronted with the unexpected, such as being disconnected from the server or having a window open with alarming messages, e.g. "fatal error". A person with aphasia needs the time to ask a tutor to explain the "unpredictable" as it is happening, as they may be unable to take notes or recall and articulate the incident at a later time.

Clinical observation of some people with aphasia indicates that they can achieve partial success in navigating the Internet by relying on the icon-based design features of Internet browsers. The navigational toolbars of the most used Internet browsers are constructed with graphical icons, which are supported with text labels. Studies on procedural assembly tasks for younger and older people compared three presentation formats: text only, illustration only, and text combined with illustration instructions. Morrell and Park (1993) found that both young and old participants made fewer errors in performance when following instructions that incorporated text supported with illustrations, rather than text-only or illustration-only instructions. Furthermore, the addition of realistic text-relevant illustrations may be helpful in translating, organising, and integrating the information included in written instructions, thereby reducing working memory and spatial demands, and enhancing comprehension (Morrell & Echt, 1996). This indicates a need to compose training instructions that use simple text, supported by realistic illustrations, which a person with aphasia will understand and be able to refer to as often as is necessary. This style of manual is available in mainstream bookshops, however people with aphasia require a very simplified version.

AIM AND DESIGN OF THE STUDY

The overall aim of this study was to develop and evaluate a specially designed Internet training package for 20 people with aphasia. There were three stages to the study. First, an aphasia-friendly self-directed learning Internet training manual was designed in collaboration with 10 volunteers with aphasia. This was then piloted with the same 10 volunteers in the second stage of the study. The results from this pilot study showed that a tutor was required to help people with aphasia learn the Internet. The main study then evaluated the success of the training programme with 20 people with aphasia using a pre-test post-test design. A no-treatment control group in which people with aphasia were tested on their Internet skills on two occasions without training, was not considered to be appropriate at this exploratory stage.

METHOD

Pilot stage

The aim of this stage of the project was to develop specialised Internet training materials that could be used as a self-directed learning guide by people with aphasia. Ten participants with aphasia volunteered to work collaboratively with the research team in the development and trialling of the training materials. To maximise accessibility for people with aphasia, it was necessary to include only the most basic of computer and Internet instructions. Using the *Aphasia Handbook* (Parr, Pound, Bing, & Long, 1999) and other aphasia-friendly resources, a set of 10 text design guidelines for people with a language disability were developed (see Table 1). These guidelines were used in the development of a self-directed aphasia-friendly Internet training manual. The training materials were based on a mainstream browser rather than a simplified browser specifically designed for people with disabilities. The choice of a mainstream browser such as Netscape Navigator or Microsoft Internet Explorer gave people with aphasia the opportunity to access the Internet on any Internet computer, rather than being restricted to a computer with specialised software. Netscape Navigator was chosen as the browser because the icons were considered to be easier to locate and recognise than those of Microsoft Internet Explorer. Although no assistive technology was used, instructions on "How to use the mouse" were included. Nine instructional modules were developed and arranged in order from simple to more complex Internet tasks. The nine Internet modules were "Know the parts of your computer", "Search for information", "Enlarge text size", "Bookmarks" (Netscape Communicator 4.7), "Go to a web address", "Exit", "Email", "Print", and "Shut-down the computer". Instructions were based on computer terminology, which is a specialised lexicon. Exposure to this language was considered essential to the training programme due to the lack of any available synonyms.

TABLE 1
Ten text design guidelines for people with a language disability

---

1. Simplify written instructions to short phrases and sentences
2. Use commonly occurring words with the emphasis on simplicity
3. Use large font (size 14–18pt)
4. Use simplified font styles (e.g., Times new roman, Comic sans MS, Arial, Verdana)
5. Format with bulleting and numbering to set out points clearly rather than embedding points in paragraphs of running prose
6. Break down instructions or lesson into clearly defined steps and then order these steps in a logical sequence from simple to more complex
7. Use generous spacing between lines of text to maximise the effect of white space
8. Use unambiguous graphics (e.g., clip-art, photos) to support the meaning of the text rather than replace text altogether
9. Align text where possible from the left margin to simplify page layout presentation
10. Use different formatting techniques to make headings and important points stand out, e.g., a change in font size, font style, colour, or the use of borders around a text selection

---

Observation of the pilot participants determined that participants failed to make progress using the Internet materials as a self-directed tool. Barriers to self-directed learning included literacy disability, lack of experience with computer hardware, in particular the mouse and keyboard, lack of computer interface experience, difficulty comprehending text instructions based on computer terminology, difficulty with visual tracking between a hardcopy manual and the computer screen, difficulty remembering the steps in the text instructions, confusion at unpredictable screen messages (e.g. "fatal error") and general anxiety with using a new technology. The participants mostly asked for assistance from the researcher in preference to using the training manual.

It was evident that people with aphasia needed a personal tutor to guide them through the training sessions. Consequently, the self-directed learning model was abandoned in favour of a hands-on tutor–student training model. The following changes to the training method and materials were implemented in response to the needs and feedback of the pilot participants.

- A tutor's instructional manual was developed to accompany the original manual.
- The original Internet tasks plus additional tasks, which had been suggested by the pilot participants, were included in both the tutor's instructional manual and the revised student manual.
- The original nine modules were reorganised into a more user-friendly sequence, beginning with the simplest tasks and moving progressively to more complex ones.
- The new design incorporated four modules that were taught over six lessons with the option of additional sessions. Lessons were designed to be between one and one and a half hours' duration.

Outcome measures

The degree of aphasia impairment would be assessed as a baseline measure, using the Western Aphasia Battery (Kertesz, 1982). Other measures developed specifically for this project are explained below.

Pre and post Internet skills assessment. This assessment was developed to measure baseline Internet skills and to provide a measure of change. The assessment measured the level of independence in 12 Internet tasks, which were covered in the nine modules. These included: "Turn on the computer", "Connect to the Internet", "Surf the net", "Do a search", "Go to a web address", "Save a site in Bookmarks/Favorites", "Exit to the desktop", "Connect to email/Read Inbox" (Outlook Express or Hotmail), and "Send an email", "Reply to an email", "Print a page", and "Shut-down the computer" A 5-point scale of independence was used to measure the level of independence reached on each Internet task, from totally independent to not at all independent.

Pre- and post-test questionnaires for the participants with aphasia. The pre-test questionnaire contained questions regarding the participants' level of education, previous computer and Internet experience, current Internet usage habits, access to Internet facilities, and attitudes to learning the Internet. The post-training questionnaire included additional questions about the Internet training intervention, e.g., if and how the training sessions had been useful, if the person had benefited from learning to use the Internet, how useful the manual had been.

Post-test questionnaire for tutors. This questionnaire included questions about Internet experience and previous tutoring experience of any kind. Other questions asked whether tutors enjoyed the experience of being an Internet tutor and whether they felt confident using the Internet training materials with their student. Tutors were asked to give feedback on the design of the training intervention and whether they would be interested in repeating this experience with another Internet student with aphasia.

MAIN STUDY

Participants

A total of 20 participants with aphasia were recruited through the Queensland University Aphasia Groups and various hospital clinics. Exclusion criteria included visual and hearing deficits that impacted on the ability to see words on a screen and hear instructions. One participant was excluded post training because of visual deficits, which became apparent during the training period. The participants included 9 women and 11 men who ranged in age from 29 to 89 years with a mean age of 59 years. Two participants had attained primary-school level education standards, eleven had completed secondary-school level, and seven participants had completed tertiary level standard. The range of aphasia duration was 1 year to 9 years with a mean of 3.1 years. Each participant was matched with a volunteer tutor.

Tutors

The 20 tutors were recruited through volunteer organisations, seniors' computer groups, stroke groups, and personal networks. They ranged in age from 14 to 74 years with a mean age of 41 years. All tutors had used the Internet from between 1 to 10 years with a mean frequency of 3.4 years. With regard to current frequency of Internet usage, 14 tutors used the Internet every day and the remaining 6 tutors used the Internet a few times a week. Of the 20 tutors, 14 said they had some previous experience of tutoring, but not necessarily in an Internet tutoring situation.

Procedure

A speech pathologist administered the Western Aphasia Battery (Kertesz, 1982). Each participant was then matched with a volunteer tutor. A member of the research team interviewed each tutor. It was essential that tutors had basic Internet experience and well-developed communication skills, and be available to volunteer their time for a minimum of six lessons. If the tutor was assessed as suitable, a convenient training venue for both the student and the tutor was arranged. Many student–tutor pairs accessed Internet facilities at a public library, which was accessible to the student. A member of the research team attended the introductory meeting of each tutor–participant pair. The purpose of this meeting was to facilitate communication between the tutor and the participant, exchange contact details, administer the pre-training assessments, confirm the dates of the training sessions, and distribute the training materials. This member of the research team was the liaison person for each tutor–participant pair throughout the training period. The liaison person contacted the participant and the tutor by phone after the first, third, and fifth sessions to check on the progress of the training programme. The participants with aphasia and the tutors were also encouraged to contact the liaison person by phone if they required support during the training intervention. At the completion of training, a researcher conducted the post-training assessments and the tutor completed the post-training questionnaire.

RESULTS

Aphasia test results

The Western Aphasia Battery (Kertesz, 1982) aphasia quotient ranged from 16.9 to 91.2 with a mean of 64.7. The WAB reading score range was 44.5 to 98 with a mean score of 71.7, and the WAB writing scores ranged from 25 to 94 with a mean of 54.7. The WAB combined reading and writing scores ranged from 8 to 18.2 with a mean of 12.6.

Aphasia typology was determined according to classifications in the Western Aphasia Battery, with six people presenting with anomic aphasia, nine with Broca's aphasia, three with conduction aphasia, and one each with Wernicke's aphasia and transcortical aphasia.

Pre and post Internet skills assessment. Participants with aphasia were rated on a 1–5 scale of independence from (1) not at all independent to (5) totally independent for 12 Internet tasks before and after the training programme. Figure 1 shows the pre and post mean ratings for all tasks. The pre-test mean score for "Turning on the computer" was 2.15 and the pre-test mean scores for the 11 remaining Internet tasks ranged from 1 to 1.8. Post-training means indicated scores between 3 and 4.1 for all tasks, with the exception of "Save a site in Bookmarks/Favorites", which resulted in a mean of 2.55.

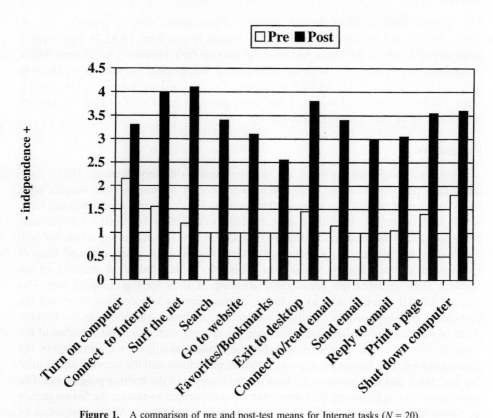

Figure 1. A comparison of pre and post-test means for Internet tasks ($N = 20$).

The Wilcoxon signed rank test showed that for all tasks, changes were significant ($p <$ .05). The means of the changes for performance (across all tasks) for each participant are plotted against the means of the post-test scores in Figure 2.

WAB scores and degree of change.   A Spearman's correlation between the mean amount of change and WAB reading scores, writing scores, and Aphasia quotient showed that there were significant correlations between the degree of change and the WAB scores ($r_s = 0.58$ with reading, 0.52 with writing, and 0.60 with AQ) following the training programme ($p < .05$).

Pre and post questionnaires for participants.   Prior to the intervention, the 20 participants had limited Internet experience, with 16 reporting they had never used the Internet and the remaining 4 reporting that they had rarely used the Internet. Eight participants said they had access to an Internet computer at the home of a friend or relative. The majority of participants ($N = 18$) thought they might benefit from learning to use the Internet, with the remaining two being uncertain about the nature or function of the Internet. Responses included, ''To help thinking'', ''To get information'', ''Talk to others on the Internet–friends, relatives'', ''Brother in the US and I'd like to talk to him'', ''I could talk to somebody else. Something else to do'', ''My work ... computer ... assistant to secretary for people'', ''I'm now need to get more information to learn to broaden horizons'', ''I like talking and I want to express. I have to learn'',   and ''Everyone is doing it. I want to know what it is all about''.

Post-training, when asked about the current frequency of Internet usage, one participant reported daily usage, fifteen participants indicated they were using the Internet 1–2 times per week, one other used the Internet 1–2 times a month, and three people reported that they rarely used the Internet. Participants were engaging in a variety of Internet activities, with email emerging as the most popular. Seven people said that they mainly used email, six people practised a variety of Internet activities including email, surfing, and finding information, four people mainly surfed the net, two people mainly looked up information, and one person declined to answer, indicating that he rarely used the Internet. Half of the participants reported that it was always easy to access an Internet

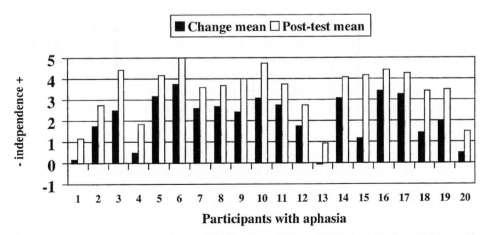

Figure 2. A comparison of the means of the changes and the means of post-test scores for participants with aphasia ($N = 20$).

computer, four said it was "mostly easy" to access an Internet computer, three participants said it was "sometimes easy", two said it was "occasionally easy" and, again, one person did not provide an answer. With regard to the intervention, eight participants said that the training sessions had been "extremely useful", seven said they were "very useful", two said "quite useful", two more said "a bit useful", and another said "not useful at all". Some of those who had said that the sessions were "useful" added the following comments: "I could keep in touch with all my family. Sending letters and photos quickly and easily", "Someone to show me through it. Over and over so it sticks", "Taught me lots of things. I can find things in it [i.e. the manual]", "We went into Caribbean [surfed] – cook[ing] tips ... printed [them]. It's fun. Tutor was very good, relaxed. Did some of the typing. Saying letters", "I like to look through the manual before I come [to the lesson]", "I said to my brother, if I got an Internet book [i.e. a mainstream text], I could never read it all to get one little bit of information. This has all of the important information is right here [in the student manual]".

Two participants said that they would have liked more lessons than the six sessions provided and three others explained why the sessions were not useful, by saying that: "I can't get to a certain point. I can't write ... reading is difficult", "[The sessions were not useful] because of my inability to decipher and understand", "I didn't understand all of it".

Participants were asked if they were able to use the student-training manual without assistance. Twelve of the twenty participants said they could use the Internet manual independently, two said they "sometimes needed help", three said they "often needed help", and three said they "always needed help". Some participants said that they no longer needed to use the manual to access the Internet: "Not really using it [now]. Used it going through programme [training period]", "I can remember by myself. Don't need it", "[The manual is] easy to follow. Good Guide". Two participants who could not use the manual independently said that there was a "Lack of time" (i.e. allotted training time is insufficient) and "It was starting [the training sessions] and I wasn't confident. I made mistakes and went backwards" (there was not enough time to absorb the information and develop Internet competency). When asked how much they had benefited from learning to use the Internet, half of the participants said "a great deal", four said "a lot", two said "somewhat", three said "a bit", and one did not provide an answer. Further comments included: "Wonderful", "It's hard [challenging]", "Able to talk to brother more often. Able to communicate with your friends on the net", "Something [all] people should be able to do. I've never done it before. At least now I can see [email] my mate at the bay. I can send an email", "[I'm] exercising my brain", "Sue [tutor] came in [taught me]. Now I can work on by myself. I won't be fully aware. I get the book and computer and day to day get better and better", "Opened up new interests for me. My daughter says I won't write a letter, but this [email] I talk every day", "Because it [the computer] doesn't consider me as stupid. If I make a mistake it just doesn't work. If I get upset, I shut it down and come back later".

When asked if they enjoyed using the Internet, seven participants responded "a great deal", seven said "a lot", five said "somewhat", and one said they enjoyed using the Internet "a bit". Participants were asked if they thought it was important for other people to learn to use the Internet, to which seven responded "extremely important", four said "very important", four said "somewhat important", another said "slightly important", and four others declined to answer to the choices provided, saying that they could not make this judgement for other people. When asked if they thought it was important for other people with aphasia to learn to use the Internet, eight participants responded "extremely important", two said "very important", three said "somewhat important", another said "slightly important", and six declined to answer to the choices provided, saying that they could not make this judgement for other people with aphasia. Participants made the following comments on the student manual: "For people who have never used it [the Internet] before, it's [the manual] really good. It's still going to take me two days to write a letter—spellcheck helps", "It's a good tool for people. It's a good skill for everybody. It's only a tool [the manual]—it's not going to get them out of the one problem [solve all problems]. The one problem is that you can't compose a message—it doesn't solve that".

Post-training questionnaire for tutors.   When asked if they had enjoyed the experience of being a tutor in this research project, fourteen tutors answered "very much", four answered "quite a lot", and two said they had "somewhat enjoyed" the experience. Further comments included: "Enjoyed sharing knowledge with others. Like to help out and to see their lives enriched with this new technology", "I learnt a lot about the Internet, for example, using favorites and history. I think you learn more when you teach someone", "Enjoyed working through the steps. Good for me to get back to basics", "I have a thirst for knowledge and hope others have, I like to pass on and make others aware of this 'information superhighway'. It's good for people to be mentally challenged", "Enjoyed being able to provide care/help for someone, made me feel good about myself", and "Getting to know someone was rewarding. You take people for granted you know. [It's a] huge resource [i.e. the Internet]. [It's a] new world for people to access", "[My student] was not catching on at the end. Feels like I am bashing my head against a brick wall. Enjoyed some parts, when he picked it up. He didn't take off with ideas about sites or addresses. Needed prompting all the time", and "I'm not cut out to be a teacher, I think I've decided".

Confidence in using the training materials was very high, with thirteen tutors saying they felt very confident, six being quite confident, and one saying they felt "somewhat confident". Tutors added the following comments: "As I mentioned earlier, I wasn't particularly familiar with the Internet, so teaching someone was a challenge, but the manual was excellent!!", "It [the manual] explained everything clearly and concisely", "[The manual was] set out logically to encompass training program in 6 sessions", "Easy step-by-step instruction. Simplified. Basics through to complicated", "Good coverage of areas to help disability such as slowing down [mouse] clicking", and "Manual covered all aspects of training, so no problems encountered". When asked if they would be prepared to repeat the experience as an Internet tutor, a majority of tutors ($N = 15$) expressed a willingness to repeat the training with another person with aphasia.

DISCUSSION

The aim of this research was to determine if people with aphasia could learn to use the Internet with the help of aphasia-friendly Internet training materials and the assistance of a voluntary tutor in a one-to-one training situation. Findings indicate that it is possible for people with aphasia to reach various levels of independence in using the Internet with the assistance of specially designed materials and a personal tutor.

The Wilcoxon signed rank test that compared the pre- and post-test ratings on Internet skills indicated that for all Internet tasks, changes were significant. The task of "Turning on the computer" was rated as the task with the highest pre-test mean at 2.15 level of independence. The post-test mean for this task (3.30) was not as high as expected because six of the twenty participants could not be rated, as they were trained and tested on network computers, some of which were permanently turned on during the training sessions and prior to the assessment. It is interesting to note that of the 14 people who could be assessed post-test, 13 scored full independence scores of 5 and one scored a 3 for moderate independence. "Shutting-down the computer" rated the second highest pre-test score for independence at 1.80. Unlike "Turning on the computer", a task that comprised one or two push-button actions, "Shutting down the computer" required participants to locate the "Start" button with the mouse, follow a series of screen instructions, and perhaps push buttons to turn off the computer. This task also rated lower than expected for post-test scores (3.6), as three of the twenty people were unable to be assessed post-test due to using networked computers. Furthermore, two more people achieved scores of 1 and 2 due to their inability to control the mouse. Of the 15 remaining participants, 13 scored 5 for full independence, and the two others scored a 1 and a 2.

The pre-test means for the remaining 10 Internet tasks ranged from 1 to 1.55. This low level of independence reflected the general lack of Internet experience in the group, with 16 participants having "never" used the Internet and 4 having used it "rarely". The lowest post-test mean score (2.55) was recorded for the task "Save a site in Bookmarks/ Favorites" ("Bookmarks" refers to Netscape Navigator and "Favorites" refers to Internet Explorer). This task appeared to be the most challenging, as it required participants to have a conceptual understanding and experience of working with Windows. It appeared that it was difficult for participants to comprehend the concept of one window being on top of another window. As this difficulty became apparent, it was decided it was necessary to include basic instructions about working with (Microsoft) Windows in module 2. The task of "Surf the net" required participants to click the mouse on hyperlinks, use scroll down buttons, click on buttons ("go"/"continue"), use drop-down menus, enter text and/or use "back"/ "forward"/ "home" buttons. Participants could do one or any combination of these steps to achieve a result, for example, some participants may have simply clicked from one hyperlink to the next (a score of 3), while others explored the full range of surfing options (a score of 4–5). Consequently it is not surprising that participants achieved the highest levels of independence on this task, as "Surfing" is less complex than tasks such as "Email". While a person with aphasia may be able to understand the function of a single icon, such as the "Back" button, they appear to have difficulty with performing a sequence of steps in an Internet task, such as "Doing a search" or "Sending an Email". This is evident in the post-test means for the three email tasks "Connect to Email and read the Inbox", "Reply to Email", "Send an Email" which resulted in scores of 3.40, 3, and 3.05 respectively. The task "Connect to the Internet" also reflected a high post-test mean of 4, once again indicating that the tasks requiring fewer steps (for this task there were two steps), are likely to place a lesser demand on working memory and cognitive and language abilities.

Although by the end of the training period, participants were engaging in all Internet activities in which they had been trained, email was the most popular choice. Enthusiasm for the Net appeared to be high at the time of post-test, with the majority of participants ($N = 15$) using the Internet once or twice per week. It is unknown whether people with aphasia sustained this degree of usage following training, without the assistance of a personal tutor. The term "digital divide" in fact can be misleading, as it suggests that "one leap and you are able to cross the chasm to eternal digital competence". The reality is that even people who do not have a disability, experience frustration at learning and continuing to use this new technology. Furthermore it is recognised that to continue to develop new skills it is essential to seek assistance. Avenues for continued support cover a range of resources including books, magazines (E-zines), online support, phone support, and the advice of friends whose knowledge exceeds one's own! Such avenues are often not available or possible for people with aphasia.

In terms of independence levels at the completion of the training period, eight of twenty participants achieved mean scores between 4 and 5, which indicated they were mostly independent. Of the twelve participants remaining, three achieved very low post-test mean scores of 1.17, 1.50, and .92 because of their continued inability to master control of the mouse. Two participants had severe apraxia and the third person had age-related motor weakness and impaired spatial awareness. The use of independence scores as a measure of success is interesting to explore further, in light of a comparison between quantitative scores for independence and qualitative feedback of participants. The experience of two participants who scored a low mean for both change and post-test scores will be discussed.

Case 1: Mary

Mary is an 89-year-old woman with Broca's aphasia who is 2 years post stroke. Mary has a WAB aphasia quotient of 33.9, a WAB reading score of 59, and a WAB writing score of 36. She lives with her son, daughter in law, and three grandchildren, one of whom is her full-time carer. Prior to her stroke, Mary was a very active and popular community member, attending her local lawn bowls club and participating in a broad range of social events. Since the stroke, she had withdrawn from face-to-face social contact with her friends because of her embarrassment regarding her aphasia. She has no expressive speech, however she has good comprehension of conversation. She has no physical disability and continues to go for her daily walk. Mary's granddaughter and carer Catherine attended and participated in all training sessions and practised with Mary between sessions. Prior to the training, Mary did not know what the Internet was. After seven training sessions, Mary remained fully dependent on her granddaughter to operate the mouse, due to fine motor weakness and age-related decline in spatial awareness. This limitation in operating the computer hardware resulted in low scores of independence. Mary scored a mean for change of 0.5 and a post-test mean of 1.50. However, despite remaining dependent on her carer, Mary was participating actively in several Internet activities. Although Mary had no expressive speech she was able to indicate her wishes to her granddaughter by gesture and yes/no responses. Being an avid sports follower and pet lover, Mary was able to ask her granddaughter to look up a range of Internet sites. She was able to look at the news, join a pet owners' club online, and follow the activities of her favourite sports stars. Most importantly, Mary was able to be in contact with her brother by email. Unlike phone communication where Mary was a passive listener, email provided a way for her to compose and send her own message with the help of her granddaughter. Online communication with some of her friends at the bowls club also helped to bypass the embarrassment she felt in face-to face communication. At the completion of training Mary was using the Internet twice a week. Despite her low levels of independence, Mary said she had benefited a great deal from learning the Internet and highly recommended it to other people with aphasia.

Case 2: Sammy

Sammy is a 54-year-old man with Broca's aphasia with a WAB aphasia quotient of 70.7, a WAB reading score of 63, and a WAB writing score of 58. Sammy is 2 years post stroke and lives with his partner. He is very sociable and copes in undemanding communication situations, however he has difficulty with more abstract and high-level concepts. He was keen to learn the Internet, saying that "I'm now need to get more information to learn to broaden my horizons." He arranged his own tutor and initiated contact between his tutor and the research team. During the training sessions it was evident that Sammy had difficulty with more abstract concepts and his tutor found it necessary to use concrete and repetitive instructions. Sammy achieved a change mean of 1.7 and post-test mean of 1.17. He said that the lessons were "very useful" but "[there] should have been more lessons". Sammy was excited about the potential of the Internet but he was also frustrated by the limitations imposed by his aphasia. He also said that he thought it was "very important" for people with aphasia to learn the Internet. Following the intervention, Sammy was persistently proactive in seeking further Internet training opportunities in a group with other people with aphasia.

In light of these two cases and other cases in this research, it must be recognised that quantitative scores convey only a partial picture of the experience of people with aphasia learning the Internet. The individual experience of participants with aphasia is more richly captured in their qualitative feedback. Indeed, although independence remains the benchmark of Internet training for the non-disability sector, it must be considered whether it is a realistic or justifiable goal to aim for within a six-lesson training pro-gramme for people with aphasia. This is especially so in the light of the obtuse nature of the digital divide, as already mentioned. Furthermore, if a person with aphasia fails to achieve full independence scores within this period, or indeed ever, does this render exposure to and training in Internet skills pointless? The qualitative feedback from participants with aphasia would strongly suggest not.

Numerous issues relating to the digital divide, and concerning people with aphasia, emerged during the pilot stage of the research and these have already been mentioned. Some training barriers, which were expected, were verified by the Spearman's correla-tion, which found that changes in Internet skills were positively correlated with the severity of the aphasia. Other less expected issues arose as the main research proceeded. For instance, it was anticipated that most people with aphasia would have ease of access to an Internet computer for the period of the training. However, only eight participants had access to an Internet computer at the home of a friend or relative. Consequently, the training schedule was held up considerably as the liaison person searched for suitable Internet training facilities. It transpired that 12 of the 20 participants were trained using networked computer systems in public libraries, school or University libraries, or seniors' organisations. Reliance on networked computers raised some unexpected problems. For example, the training manuals had originally been designed using Netscape navigator 4.7. However the public library system was networked with the browser Microsoft Internet Explorer. Consequently, another complete version of the training manuals had to be created for Internet Explorer 5.5. Email posed another problem, as the program included in the materials was Outlook Express and this was not an option in public libraries. A decision was made to create a training module for Hotmail, as this would allow people to send and receive their mail on any Internet computer rather than just the one with the Outlook Express program. Thus participants had a choice: they could choose either Outlook Express or Hotmail. Outlook Express was recommended if they were using their own computer, otherwise Hotmail was preferable.

Other issues that emerged as a result of training in libraries were transport issues to and from the library, waiting times to reserve Internet computers, and background noise and activity compromising the ability of participants to concentrate and communicate. A positive outcome resulting from the library training was that participants became aware of the existence of Internet facilities at their local library and this provided them with the opportunity of continuity of Internet access following the training period. Library training introduced the participants to a new venue and new faces and in general most librarians were very welcoming and encouraging about the training initiative and providing ongoing support.

One unexpected issue that arose during the recruitment of tutors was the lack of availability of volunteers within family and friend networks. Surprisingly, only two tutors were in these categories. One participant was tutored by his sister and another by a friend. Tutors were mostly difficult to recruit from family and friend networks because of lack of time and availability. The remaining 18 tutors were recruited through a volunteer organisation, the university student network, and seniors' Internet organisations. This placed an unexpected strain on resources as the research team advertised, interviewed, and screened prospective tutors over a wide geographical area, then matched them to a suitable participant, and finally organised Internet training facilities, which had to be accessible to both parties. Hence Internet training for people with aphasia is not without resource implications, even when community tutors and community venues are used.

Overall, the experience appears to have been satisfying for tutors, with the majority saying that they enjoyed the experience "very much" and "quite a lot". The training materials themselves appear to have been accessible and easy to use, with 13 tutors saying they were "very confident" using the training materials. The feedback of tutors in the development of the training materials was extremely useful and the importance of the selection of appropriate tutors to deliver the training materials cannot be overstated. Quite simply the programme relies heavily on the strong communication skills and personal qualities of tutors to successfully deliver the training materials to people with aphasia.

The accessibility of the student manual to the participants with aphasia was assessed with the question "Are you able to use the manual by yourself?". Twelve participants said they could use the manual independently. This does not mean that they could complete Internet tasks independently, but rather that they could use their manual as a guide whilst sitting at the computer, without asking for assistance in interpreting the instructions. Not surprisingly, levels of independence with using the manual varied greatly within the group, with three participants saying they always needed someone's help. Enthusiasm for the Internet was high at the end of training with 14 people saying they had benefited "a great deal" or "a lot" from the intervention. Similarly, 14 participants said they enjoyed using the Internet "a great deal" or "a lot". Furthermore, half of the participants said that it was either "extremely important" or "very important" for people with aphasia to learn to use the Internet.

A perceived limitation of the quantitative aspects of the study might be the reliability and validity of the assessments used. The assessment tool comprising twelve Internet tasks was developed to measure how independently participants completed discrete Internet tasks. While an attempt was made to break each task into linear steps, there are times when Internet tasks may be executed in different ways. Therefore, while pre-test interrater reliability of two researchers was at 77.27%, there were times that further reliability checks were performed due to the unexpected responses of participants; consequently, it is possible that reliability factors may have impacted slightly on the quantitative results.

This paper has identified and attempted to address digital divide issues for people with aphasia. The barriers are numerous and complex, and although this type of research is a digression from mainstream speech pathology research, it is important to note the essential role of speech pathologists in the development of such materials. The training materials have been developed in collaboration with people with aphasia and a set of 10 text design guidelines for people with a language disability has been proposed.

In conclusion, results from this research have been encouraging. People with aphasia have been able to achieve varying degrees of success in learning to use the Internet. This has been achieved using specially designed materials and the assistance of one-to-one tutoring. It has also been concluded that independence, as a benchmark for success, is not always a valid goal for this particular group of people. The training materials used in this project have been designed to be accessible to people with aphasia, however their broad application to other groups of people with language, cognitive, and literacy disabilities is evident. Further research on the effectiveness of the training programme for groups of people with traumatic brian injury and Parkinson's disease is forthcoming. The training manuals are available as a free download at

http://www.shrs.uq.edu.au/cdaru/aphasiagroups/

REFERENCES

A strategic framework for the information economy (2001). National Office of the Information Economy. Retrieved 10/02/02, from the World Wide Web: *http://www.noie.gov.au/projects/access/community/digi-taldivide/Digitaldivide.htm*

Clothier, P. (1996). *The complete computer trainer.* New York: McGraw-Hill.

Commonwealth Disability Strategy (2001). Retrieved 12/3/02, from the World Wide Web: *http://www.facs.-gov.au/disability/cds/cds/outcomes.htm*

Echt, K. V., Morrell, R. W., & Park, D. C. (1998). Effects of age and training formats on basic computer skill acquisition in older adults. *Educational Gerontology, 24,* 3–25.

Egan, J., & Worrall, L. (2001). *Queensland University Aphasia Groups. University of Queensland.* Retrieved 17/3/02, from the World Wide Web: *http://dexter.shrs.uq.edu.au/cdaru/aphasiagroups/*

Elman, R. J. (2001). The Internet and aphasia: Crossing the digital divide. *Aphasiology, 15*(10/11), 895–899.

Jordan, L., & Kaiser, W. (1996). *Aphasia—A social approach* (1st Ed.). London: Chapman & Hall.

Kaye, H. S. (2000). *Computer and Internet use among people with disabilities. (Disability Statistics Report 13).* San Francisco: California University.

Kertesz, A. (1982). *The Western Aphasia Battery.* San Antonio, CA: The Psychological Corporation.

Morrell, R. W., & Echt, K. V. (1996). Instructional design for older computer users: The influence of cognitive factors. In W. A. Rogers (Ed.), *Aging and skilled performance: Advances in theory application* (pp. 241–265). Hillsdale, NJ: Lawrence Erlbaum Associates Inc.

Morrell, R. W., & Park, D. C. (1993). The effects of age, illustrations, and task variables on the performance of procedural assembly tasks. *Psychology and Aging, 8,* 389–399.

Owens, J., Lamb, G., & Keller, S. (2001). *Literature review of computer and Internet training for people with disabilities.* Melbourne: Deakin University.

Parr, S., Pound, C., Bing, S., & Long, B. (1999). *The aphasia handbook.* London: Connect Press.

Peng, R., Adams, L. A., & Gentile, A. (1998). Conquering community barriers: Stroke rehabilitation. In W. Sife (Ed.), *After stroke: Enhancing quality of life* (pp. 233–246). New York: The Haworth Press Inc.

Pillay, H. (2000). *Technology uptake scrutinised. Queensland University of Technology.* Retrieved 15/3/02, from the World Wide Web: *http://www.qut.edu.au/chan/corpcomm/site/archives/apr2000/iqstory25.html*

Riviere, C. N., & Thakor, N. V. (1996). Effects of age and disability on tracking tasks with a computer mouse: Accuracy and linearity. *Journal of Rehabilitation Research and Development, 33*(1), 6–14.

Stoddard, S., & Nelson, J. (2001). Math, computer and the Internet: Better employment opportunities for persons with disabilities. *American Rehabilitation, 26*(6), 1–9.

The World Wide Web Consortium (2001). Retrieved 13/07/03, from the World Wide Web: *http://www.w3.org/*

Website found to be discriminatory (2000). Richard Pryor & Associates Commercial lawyers. Retrieved 27/7/03, from the World Wide Web: *http://www.pryor.com.au/socog.htm*

Index